Praise for
WaLKiNG L.a.

"*Walking L.A.* is a must-have for Angelenos and tourists alike . . . Get your hands
on a copy of this hot little book immediately and go wild."

—Gloria Lintermans, *Retro Chic*

" . . . if you learn one thing from *Walking L.A.*, it's that a neighborhood
doesn't have to be ritzy or a tourist hub to merit the expenditure
of shoe leather and a leisurely hour or two."

—*Daily News*

"*Walking L.A.* takes you on dozens of walking tours
to explore places right under your nose."

—ABC7 Eyewitness News

"Throughout her book, [Erin Mahoney Harris] points out parts of
Los Angeles that many people may not know about."

—KCET's *Life & Times*

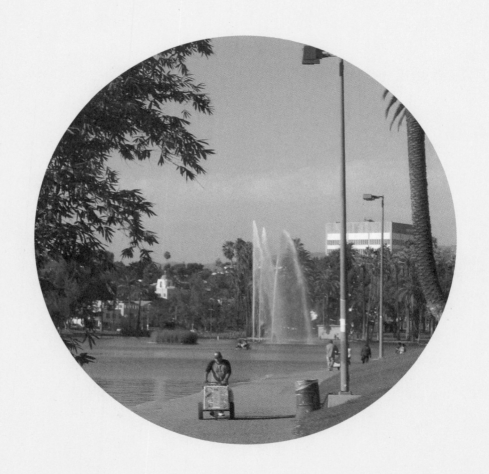

WALKING
L.a.

38 walking tours exploring stairways, streets, and buildings you never knew existed

SECOND EDITION

Erin Mahoney Harris

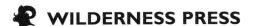 **WILDERNESS PRESS**

Walking L.A.: 38 walking tours exploring stairways, streets, and buildings you never knew existed

1st EDITION October 2005
2nd EDITION May 2008
   3rd printing 2014

Copyright © 2005, 2008 by Erin Mahoney Harris

Cover photos copyright © 2008 by Erin Mahoney Harris
Interior photos: Erin Mahoney Harris
Maps: Bart Wright, Lohnes+Wright
Book and cover design and layout: Larry B. Van Dyke
Book editor: Eva Dienel

ISBN 978-0-89997-471-2

Manufactured in the United States of America

Published by: **Wilderness Press**
                c/o Keen Communications
                P.O. Box 43673
                Birmingham, AL 35243
                www.wildernesspress.com
Visit our website for a complete listing of our books and for ordering information.

Distributed by Publishers Group West

Cover photos: *Front, clockwise from bottom center:* The bluffs in Santa Monica, Buster's in South Pasadena, La Brea Tar Pits, George Stanley Fountain, Los Angeles City Hall, Chateau Marmont
Back, clockwise from bottom left: Los Angeles Theatre, walking in South Pasadena, Brand Library & Art Center
Frontispiece: Echo Park Lake

acknowledgments

The call for me to create a second edition of this book came during an especially busy and exciting period in my life, as I had just given birth to my first child. I'm grateful to have had so much support from my husband, Tony Harris, who has always had profound faith in my abilities. The fact that my mother, Ann Mahoney, is an English teacher sometimes felt like the bane of my existence when I was a student, but I now realize how fortunate I was to have a writing tutor with such a heavy personal investment in my future. I was also fortunate enough to marry into a family of exceptional people, and have enjoyed the love and encouragement of John and Marjorie Harris and Gloria Lintermans. Finally, I'd like to thank West Donovan Harris for adding an amazing new dimension to my life and for sleeping quietly in his stroller while Mommy did research for her book.

author's note

The face of Los Angeles is constantly changing, particularly when it comes to residential and commercial architecture, so you may find on your journeys that certain landmarks and features described in this book have changed since it was written. I encourage you to use my directions as a general guide, but to explore each neighborhood at a leisurely pace and make your own discoveries. That said, I also implore you to use common sense on your walks to ensure your safety and comfort: Bring a buddy if you're exploring a new neighborhood that you don't feel entirely at ease about visiting; take your walks during the day rather than at night; wear appropriate shoes to prevent blisters; if you bring your dog along, keep him/her on a leash at all times, as these are primarily urban routes in close proximity to street traffic; and, finally, if you're bringing a baby or child in a stroller on your walk, please pay attention to the difficulty rating to see if stairways are part of that route. (Please be aware that those routes that have only a few steps here and there do not include the stairway notation.)

The boundaries mentioned at the beginning of each walk are meant to give you an idea of the major streets that surround the route in order to make it easier to find. These streets do not always appear on the accompanying maps, so please refer to the Thomas Guide coordinates provided or a separate map if you have trouble locating the start of a walk. For those walks located within a mile of a Metro station, I've included that information as well.

Happy trekking!

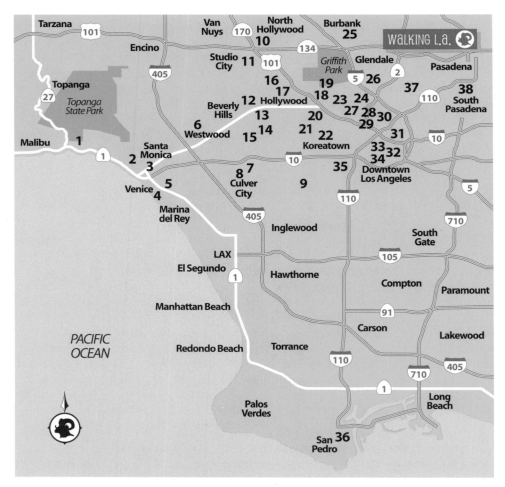

Numbers on this locator map correspond to Walk numbers.

TaBLe OF CONTeNTS

INTRODUCTION

Los Angeles has gotten a bad rap.

Sure, it's sprawling, traffic-choked, and smoggy. Its public transportation system leaves a lot to be desired, and the old adage that it takes 20 minutes to drive anywhere in the city is woefully misleading.

But it is a great place to walk. Really, it is—don't be deterred by the maze of freeways and pervasive car culture. No, you won't be able to traverse the greater metro area in a day, or even in a weekend, but take it in smaller doses, and you'll be rewarded with a deeper understanding of this city's unique blend of culture, architecture, and topography.

For the second edition of this book, I have expanded the boundaries of the first to include cities and neighborhoods I find especially charming, such as family-friendly South Pasadena and Glendale's Kenneth Village, which has a delightful small-town feel. This edition also includes additions to make it even easier for readers to explore the city on foot, such as information about nearby Metro station stops and notes about which walks include stairways (especially useful for stroller-pushers like myself). Finally, this edition has a whole slew of new points of interest, as well as four completely new routes.

The purpose of this book is to prove that walking in LA can be immensely rewarding, opening your eyes to hidden pockets of the city that you never knew existed. These walks reflect the many faces of Los Angeles, and I hope the discoveries you make as you explore the vibrant neighborhoods dotting the hills, valleys, and flatlands of this fascinating city will encourage you to dust off your sneakers and leave the car in the garage at every opportunity.

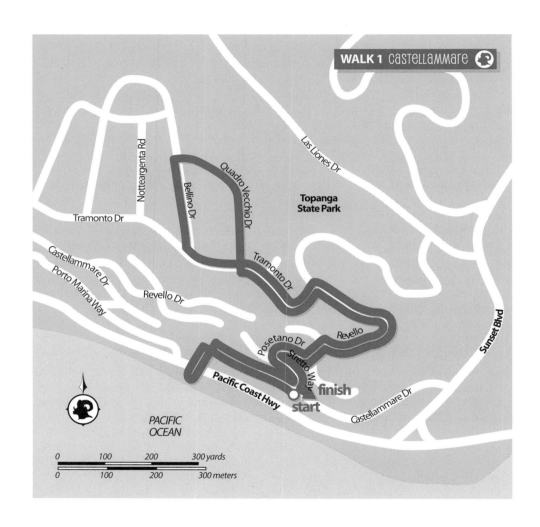

Notteargenta Rd

Quadro Vecchio Dr

Bellino Dr

Las Liones Dr

**Topanga
State Park**

Tramonto Dr

Tramonto Dr

Castellammare Dr

Porto Marina Way

Revello Dr

Posetano Dr

Revello

Stretto Way

Sunset Blvd

Pacific Coast Hwy

Castellammare Dr

finish

start

*PACIFIC
OCEAN*

0	100	200	300 yards
0	100	200	300 meters

1 castellammare: pacific palisades' "castle on the sea"

BOUNDARIES: Pacific Coast Highway, Sunset Blvd., Topanga State Park, Surfview Dr.
THOMAS GUIDE COORDINATES: Map 630; G6
DISTANCE: Approx. 1¼ miles
DIFFICULTY: Strenuous (includes stairways)
PARKING: Free street parking is available on Castellammare Dr.

This whimsically named neighborhood in the Pacific Palisades lies just east of the Pacific Coast Highway and just south of Sunset Blvd.—talk about exclusive real estate! Castellammare's lucky residents enjoy the soothing breezes and sweeping panoramas of the Pacific Ocean from their vantage point high in the hills. Of all the architecturally diverse regions in the greater Los Angeles area, this may represent the best example of the structural incongruity that so annoyed Woody Allen's character in *Annie Hall*. After all, when money is no object, people tend to go nuts building their dream homes. As you might expect on streets with names like Posetano and Tremonto, many of the homes are Mediterranean style, but you'll also find a surprising preponderance of traditional, ranch-style, and modern houses in this quietly exclusive coastal enclave.

● Begin on Castellammare Dr., just southeast of Stretto Way, and walk northwest on Castellammare, past Stretto. At 17501, stop to admire the gorgeous Spanish-style home—it's pale yellow with pretty blue trim and lots of colorful tile work. This stunner is purportedly the former abode of John Barrymore. Right next door is another Mediterranean-style home with elegantly carved wood trim; sunset views afforded by the row of windows on the second floor must be breathtaking.

● When you reach the dead end, continue on the dirt path that begins to the left of the wood barrier, and pass between low trees, shrubs, and ice plant. Continue straight ahead on Castellammare where the paved street begins once again.

Just past 17560 Castellammare Dr., look for a concrete path/stairway on your left. This leads to an overpass that crosses PCH and takes you down to the beach. Head down to sink your feet into the sand and splash around in the surf. After you've had your fun, return to Castellammare via the same overpass.

- Retrace your steps on Castellammare Dr. to head across the dirt footpath and all the way back to the breathtaking Spanish home at the corner of Stretto Way.

- Turn left on Stretto Way, following the road as it curves sharply to the left. When you reach Posetano Rd., check out the three-story Italian villa climbing the hill at 17531 Posetano. In 1935, screen siren Thelma Todd died here of carbon monoxide poisoning, either by her own hand or someone else's—the mystery has never been solved. A sign above the garage declares CASTILLO DEL MAR, and this mansion indeed looks like it belongs in a neighborhood known as Castellammare.

- Turn right on Posetano Rd. Ahead, at 17437 Posetano Rd., is a striking modern home constructed of stucco, steel, glass, and wood. This is an excellent example of California-born architect Pierre Koenig's work, which uses exposed steel and glass to dramatic effect.

NearBY aND NOTaBLe

The Self-Realization Fellowship's gorgeous flagship Lake Shrine Temple, located at 17190 Sunset Blvd. about 0.3 mile north of Sunset's intersection with Castellammare Dr., is absolutely worth a visit. The lake and surrounding gardens provide numerous spots to sit and meditate, or simply to enjoy the peaceful, lush surroundings. The ornate temple overlooking the grounds blends Eastern and Western architectural styles to stunning effect. The gardens, lake, and visitor's center are open to the public Tuesday through Sunday; call 310-454-4114 for visiting hours. (To learn more about the Self-Realization Fellowship, see Walk 37.)

- Look for the stairs on your left just before 17445 and ascend them. This stairway is clean and well maintained, vibrantly bordered on the right with bougainvillea, which is abundant throughout this walk.

- At the top of the steps, turn right on Revello Dr., which is a private road for a short stretch. Many of the homes on Revello are sleek and modern in design. Follow the road as it curves to the left.

- Bear left at the intersection to follow Tramonto Dr., and pause to admire the hills of Topanga State Park on your right. As you continue along Tramonto, you'll notice an abundance of traditional-style houses, which provide a stark contrast to the sleek, modern homes on Revello. An awesome panoramic view of the Pacific opens up on your left; stop here to watch the sailboats cruising through Santa Monica Bay.

- Turn right on Quadro Vecchio Dr., a blissfully domestic street lined with ranch-style homes that couldn't look less Italian. Follow Quadro Vecchio as it curves to the left.

- Turn left on Bellino Dr., which takes you back to Tramonto Dr.

- Turn left on Tramonto, and then retrace your steps to the intersection with Revello Dr.

- Bear right at the intersection to head back along Revello Dr. Straight ahead is a great view of the Santa Monica beaches. After following the curve in the road, descend the staircase you climbed earlier.

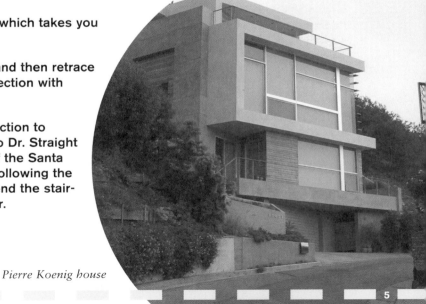

Pierre Koenig house

- Turn right on Posetano Rd. at the bottom of the stairs.

- Turn left on Stretto Way and follow the road as it curves back toward Castellammare Dr.

- Turn left on Castellammare to return to your starting point.

route summary

1. Begin on Castellammare Dr., just southwest of Sunset Blvd. and head uphill on Castellammare.

2. Continue straight ahead on the dirt path to the left of the dead end, and then continue straight on Castellammare when the paved road begins again.

3. Follow the stairs on your left to the overpass that takes you down to the beach, and then return to Castellammare Dr. via the same route.

4. Retrace your steps on Castellammare Dr., across the dirt path.

5. Turn left on Stretto Way, following the road as it curves sharply to the left.

6. Turn right on Posetano Rd.

7. Ascend the staircase on your left just before 17445 Posetano.

8. Turn right on Revello Dr. at the top of the steps.

9. Bear left at the intersection to follow Tramonto Dr.

10. Turn right on Quadro Vecchio Dr.

11. Turn left on Bellino Dr.

12. Turn left on Tramonto, and then retrace your steps back to the intersection with Revello Dr.

13. Bear right at the intersection to head back along Revello Dr., and then descend the staircase you climbed earlier.

14. Turn right on Posetano Rd. at the bottom of the stairs.

15. Turn left on Stretto Way and follow the road as it curves back toward Castellammare Dr.

16. Turn left on Castellammare Dr. to return to your starting point .

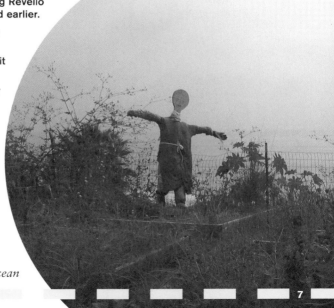

Castellammare garden overlooking the ocean

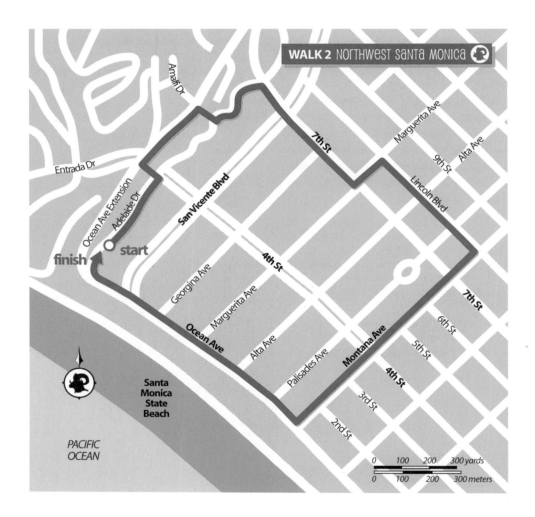

WALK 2 NORTHWEST SANTA MONICA

Amalfi Dr

7th St

Marguerita Ave

9th St

Alta Ave

Entrada Dr

Lincoln Blvd

Ocean Ave Extension

Adelaide Dr

San Vicente Blvd

4th St

start

finish

Georgina Ave

Marguerita Ave

7th St

6th St

Ocean Ave

Alta Ave

Montana Ave

5th St

Palisades Ave

4th St

Santa
Monica
State
Beach

3rd St

2nd St

PACIFIC
OCEAN

0   100   200   300 yards
0   100   200   300 meters

2 Northwest Santa Monica: rarefied air North of Montana ave.

BOUNDARIES: Ocean Ave., Entrada Dr., Lincoln Blvd., Montana Ave.
THOMAS GUIDE COORDINATES: Map 671; C1
DISTANCE: Approx. 2 miles
DIFFICULTY: Moderate (includes stairways)
PARKING: Free street parking is available on Adelaide Dr.

The northernmost reaches of Santa Monica are where you'll find some of the most outrageously priced homes in all of Los Angeles County. And it's no surprise, as this area has it all: the beach, nearby hiking trails, a good school district, and proximity to excellent places to eat and shop. This walk heads up and down Santa Monica's notoriously steep pair of Adelaide Dr. staircases before going over to Montana Ave., Santa Monica's premier shopping and dining district. It then drops down to the beach for a quick detour before returning to the starting point.

Finding the beginning of this walk can be a little tricky, as Adelaide Dr. isn't clearly marked with a street sign. As you approach the northwest end of Ocean Ave., look for two streets branching off to the right. Turn on the first street (the one that heads uphill), and you're on Adelaide. Park on the right side of the street, paying attention to posted parking enforcement signs.

- Begin by walking east on Adelaide Dr., away from the ocean. Adelaide serves as the northeast border between Santa Monica and the city of Los Angeles; the neighborhood appropriately named Rustic Canyon lies on the other side. On your right are gorgeous, multimillion-dollar homes—stately traditional houses of dark-stained wood alongside Spanish mansions. The sprawling shingled Craftsman at 236 Adelaide is particularly envy-inducing.

- At the intersection of 4th St. and Adelaide, descend the long, steep stairway on your left all the way down to Entrada Dr. The word's out about this stairway and the one you're about to climb, so you may have to yield to the remarkably fit locals doggedly trotting up and down.

- Turn right at the bottom of the steps, passing a school on your left before you reach the next set of stairs, opposite the intersection with Amalfi Dr. Ascend the long wooden staircase, again watching out for exercise addicts on their quest for buns of steel.

- Turn left at the top of the stairs, continuing along Adelaide. As you approach the intersection with 7th St., notice the unique, pueblo-style home up ahead on your right.

- Turn right on 7th St., passing a sign indicating the official Santa Monica city limits, or as some locals wryly call it, "the People's Republic of Santa Monica." After one block, cross San Vicente Blvd., which is divided by a wide meridian planted with coral trees. This is a popular path for joggers. It seems that everyone in Santa Monica is into some form of physical activity, be it jogging, biking, or stair-climbing. Continue southwest on 7th, passing an interesting architectural mix of homes—contemporary, traditional, Spanish, and Tudor.

- Turn left on Marguerita Ave. and follow it for one block to Lincoln Blvd. An impressive, shingled, Cape Cod-style house sits on the southwest corner of Marguerita and Lincoln.

- Turn right on Lincoln Blvd. At the intersection with Alta Ave., look toward the southeast corner to see an interesting modern yellow stucco home with an abundance of small windows. Continue on Lincoln past the elementary school on your left.

- Turn right on Montana Ave. This street—featuring a collection of upscale boutiques, fine restaurants, neighborhood coffeehouses, and chic spas and salons on the stretch between 7th and 17th streets—is a popular destination for the well-to-do residents of north Santa Monica. You may want to explore for a few blocks to the east before heading west back toward the ocean. Just east of the intersection with Lincoln is Cafe Boulangerie, a large bakery that now shares its space with a Panda Express.

This is unfortunate, as the scent of fresh-baked bread is now stifled by the aroma of Chinese fast-food.

● Continue west on Montana, passing the Massage Place, an affordable massage center, at 625 Montana Ave. Follow Montana Ave. for about a half mile toward the ocean through a mostly residential area.

● Once you reach Ocean Ave., cross the street and turn right to head northeast for another half mile along the greenway known as Palisades Park (or, more informally, "the bluffs"), passing a collection of high-rise condos on your right. This exclusive real estate provides an interesting juxtaposition with the many homeless who choose to sleep at Palisades Park due to the temperate climate and Santa Monica's relative tolerance for the indigent.

● As you approach the intersection with Adelaide, notice a striking white structure overlooking the sea at 101 Ocean Ave. Once you reach Adelaide, turn right and walk back up the hill to your starting point.

The bluffs

POINTS OF INTEREST

Cafe Boulangerie 804 Montana Ave., Santa Monica, CA 90403, 310-451-4998
Massage Place and Petit Spa 625 Montana Ave., Santa Monica, CA 90403, 310-393-7007

route summary

1. Begin by walking east on Adelaide Dr., away from Ocean Ave.
2. At the intersection of 4th St. and Adelaide, descend the stairway on your left to Entrada Dr.
3. Turn right at the bottom of the steps, and then climb the stairs on your right, opposite the intersection with Amalfi Dr.
4. Turn left at the top of the stairs, continuing along Adelaide.
5. Turn right on 7th St.
6. Turn left on Marguerita Ave.
7. Turn right on Lincoln Blvd.
8. Turn right on Montana Ave.
9. Continue west on Montana for about a half mile.
10. Cross Ocean Ave. and turn right.
11. Turn right on Adelaide to return to your starting point.

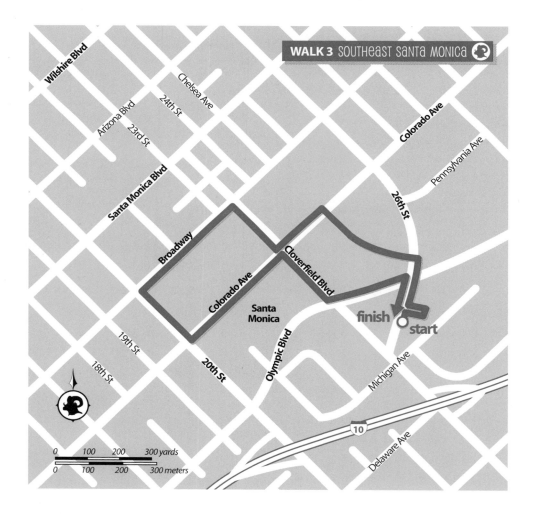

Wilshire Blvd

Chelsea Ave

24th St

Arizona Blvd

23rd St

Santa Monica Blvd

Colorado Ave

Pennsylvania Ave

26th St

Broadway

Colorado Ave

Cloverfield Blvd

Santa Monica

finish

start

19th St

18th St

20th St

Olympic Blvd

Michigan Ave

10

Delaware Ave

0   100   200   300 yards
0   100   200   300 meters

3 SOUTHEAST SANTA MONICA: MIXING BUSINESS WITH PLEASURE

BOUNDARIES: **26th St., Broadway, 20th St., 10 Freeway**
THOMAS GUIDE COORDINATES: **Map 631; H7**
DISTANCE: **Approx. 1 mile**
DIFFICULTY: **Easy**
PARKING: **Metered street parking is available on 26th St.**

When most people think of Santa Monica, they have visions of sun-kissed locals jogging along the waterfront and tourists in wide-brimmed hats and flip-flops strolling along the pier. But a couple of miles inland, it's anything but the beach. Santa Monica is also home to several colossal office parks, teeming with high-powered executives in button-down shirts and ties. This walk explores the beachside city's multimillion-dollar business development, the Water Garden, as well as Bergamot Station, a sprawling collection of art galleries occupying a former train depot hidden between the 10 Freeway and Olympic Blvd.

● Begin on 26th St. between Cloverfield Blvd. and Olympic Blvd. and head northeast on 26th, toward Olympic.

● On your right, immediately before Olympic, is the rear entrance to Bergamot Station. Allow some time to wander this maze of brick and corrugated-metal buildings, most of which house art galleries, museums, and studios. The Santa Monica Museum of Art resides at Bergamot Station, along with notable galleries such as the Shoshana Wayne, Track 16, and the Gallery of Functional Art. You can also grab a bite at the Gallery Cafe—or you can wait to take advantage of the many other opportunities to nosh on this walk.

● Exit Bergamot Station the same way you came in and continue along 26th St. to the corner of Olympic Blvd.

● Cross Olympic, and then cross 26th St. so that you are on the same side of the street as the Water Garden office complex—the one with the lovely circular fountain on the corner. Follow the perimeter of the fountain around to the point where it spills into a rivulet, and then follow the stream into the heart of the Water Garden, where it opens up into the vast collection of pools for which the complex is named.

- Continue through the courtyard, roughly following the same path as the water, which is crisscrossed with bridges and punctuated with fountains, elaborately constructed pools, and planters brimming with vibrant flowers. The Water Garden is a great place to stop and have a sandwich or a cool drink; there are tables and chairs with umbrellas all over the plaza. Unfortunately, the peaceful atmosphere is corrupted somewhat by the imposing tinted-glass and concrete office buildings rising on all sides.

- When you come to the end of the last pool, there are several eateries that cater to the weekday suit-and-tie set on your right, including Bizou Garden Bistro. After passing the final circular fountain at the entrance to the plaza, turn left on Colorado Ave. and head toward Cloverfield Blvd.

- Turn right on Cloverfield and walk one block to Broadway.

- Turn left on Broadway, and notice the colorful graffiti-art-covered building on the southwest corner. Continue west on Broadway for about a quarter mile. An unprepossessing gray stucco building at 2112 Broadway turns out to be the home of Playboy Studio West. The Lowe Gallery resides at 2034 Broadway, although you may be art-galleried-out after your visit to Bergamot Station. At 2024, you'll come to Back on Broadway, a pleasant, casual eatery offering tasty sandwiches, salads, and bakery items. This is a good place to stop in for some sustenance if you haven't already picnicked at the Water Garden.

- Turn left on 20th St. The Santa Monica Dog and Cat Hospital sits on the southeast corner.

- Walk for one block to Colorado Ave. and turn left. On the south side of the street is the enormous, rose-colored sandstone Universal/Sony Music complex. Next door to Universal/Sony is the Plaza at the Arboretum, one of those newfangled, multiuse, commercial/residential developments complete with a selection of casual dining establishments and, naturally, a Starbucks.

- At the intersection of Colorado and Cloverfield Blvd., notice the giant Universal globe teetering on its pedestal on the southwest corner. Turn right on Cloverfield and continue for one block to Olympic Blvd., passing a Ralph's grocery store on your right.

- Turn left on Olympic, crossing Cloverfield. Don't cross Olympic, as there is no sidewalk on the south side of the street. Continue along Olympic for one block; you'll see the Water Garden on your left.

- Turn right on 26th St., returning to the start of you walk.

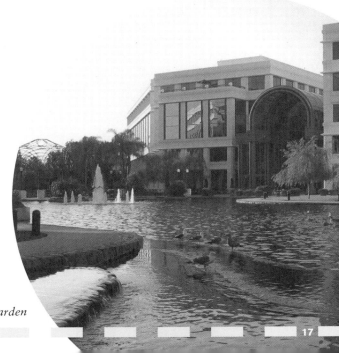

The Water Garden

POINTS OF INTEREST

Bergamot Station 2525 Michigan Ave., Santa Monica, CA 90404, 310-829-5854
Bizou Garden Bistro 2450 Colorado Ave., Santa Monica, CA 90404, 310-582-8203
Lowe Gallery 2034 Broadway, Santa Monica, CA 90404, 310-449-0184
Back on Broadway 2024 Broadway, Santa Monica, CA 90404, 310-453-8919

route summary

1. Begin on 26th St. between Cloverfield Blvd. and Olympic Blvd. and head northeast on 26th St. toward Olympic Blvd.

2. Enter Bergamot Station on the right side of the street.

3. Exit Bergamot Station the same way you went in and continue on 26th toward Olympic.

4. Cross Olympic Blvd. and then cross 26th St. so that you're on the same corner as the Water Garden office complex.

5. Cross through the Water Garden courtyard, roughly following the same path as the waterway.

6. Exit the Water Garden complex and turn left on Colorado Ave.

7. Turn right on Cloverfield Blvd.

8. Turn left on Broadway.

9. Turn left on 20th St.

11. Turn left on Colorado Ave.

12. Turn right on Cloverfield Blvd.

13. Turn left on Olympic Blvd.

14. Turn right on 26th St. to return to your starting point.

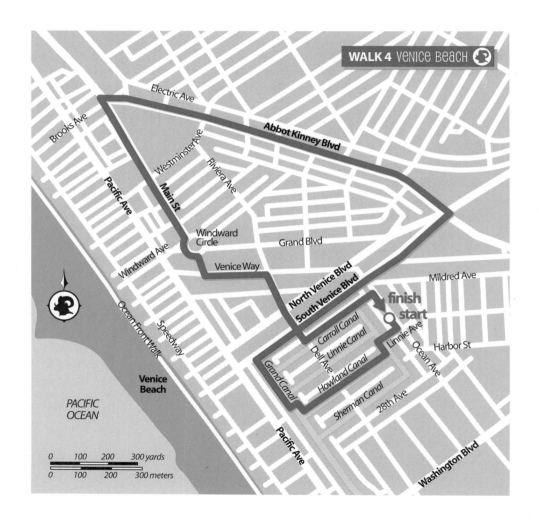

Electric Ave

Brooks Ave

Abbot Kinney Blvd

Pacific Ave

Westminster Ave

Riviera Ave

Main St

Windward Circle

Grand Blvd

Windward Ave

Venice Way

North Venice Blvd

South Venice Blvd

Mildred Ave

finish
start

Ocean Front Walk

Speedway

Carroll Canal

Dell Ave

Linnie Canal

Linnie Ave

Ocean Ave

Harbor St

Grand Canal

Howland Canal

Sherman Canal

28th Ave

Washington Blvd

Venice Beach

PACIFIC OCEAN

Pacific Ave

0   100   200   300 yards
0   100   200   300 meters

4 Venice Beach:
Old World Italy Meets
Funky Socal Beach Culture

BOUNDARIES: **Abbot Kinney Blvd., Pacific Ave., Washington Blvd.**
THOMAS GUIDE COORDINATES: **Map 671; H6**
DISTANCE: **Approx. 2 miles**
DIFFICULTY: **Easy**
PARKING: **Free street parking is available on Ocean Ave.**

Venice Beach is probably the most distinctive beach town in all of Southern California, made all the more unique by its charming canals, which were built by Abbot Kinney in 1904 as an homage to the city's forebear in Italy. Here you'll find none of the snootiness that you might encounter in Malibu or Palos Verdes; Venice is more funky than fussy. That's not to say that the people who live here, particularly in the neighborhoods that line the canals and the ocean-front, aren't affluent. But Venice is still more affordable than next-door Santa Monica, and one might argue that it has a good deal more personality, as well.

Note: This walk can be particularly fun for both you and your pooch, provided he doesn't get overexcited at the sight of ducks. If you do bring him, resist the temptation to remove his leash during the canal portion of the walk. Toward the end of the route, you'll come to the Westminster off-leash dog park, where Rover can get footloose and fancy-free with his canine pals.

- **This excursion begins in the South Venice neighborhood, just south of Venice Blvd. Begin by walking south on Ocean Ave. toward Linnie Ave. Notice that the houses along this stretch of Ocean are all relatively modest in size and style—some even have the appearance of one-room shacks.**

- **Turn right on Linnie Ave.**

- Cross the bridge arching over the Eastern Canal, pausing on top to admire the interesting mix of homes lining the waterway. The houses here are decidedly grander than those on Ocean Ave., ranging in architectural style from American Colonial Revival to modern to Tudor Revival.

- On the other side of the bridge, make an immediate left to follow the sidewalk along the canal.

- Follow the sidewalk as it turns to the right, taking you along Howland Canal. Ducks are everywhere, quackily going about their business, and small boats and canoes are parked at mini-docks in front of some houses. The homes along this waterway are all beautifully maintained and each is distinct. Notable architectural styles here include Craftsman, Spanish Colonial Revival, Cape Cod, and modern stucco beach homes with huge picture windows.

- Cross Dell Ave. and then pause in the shade of the giant pine tree to bask in the tranquil, salt-tinged air of this remarkable neighborhood. It's hard not to envy the residents and their Old-World-Italy-meets-funky-SoCal-beach-culture lifestyle. Unlike in most Los Angeles neighborhoods, homes are rarely for sale in this area.

- Follow the sidewalk as it turns right at the corner of Grand Canal.

- Cross the pedestrian bridge on your left and then turn right to continue along the walkway on the other side of Grand Canal. You'll pass a canoe rental facility on the left.

- Follow the pedestrian walkway up to South Venice Blvd. and turn right. The Venice Farmers Market sets up in the parking lot on the northeast corner of Dell Ave. and South Venice Blvd. every Friday from 7 to 11 A.M.

- Continue on South Venice Blvd. for a little less than a half mile to Abbot Kinney Blvd.

- Turn left on Abbot Kinney.

- Continue along Abbot Kinney for three quarters of a mile. If you're in the mood for shopping, you'll be pleased to find vintage clothing, chic couture, art, furniture, surfboards, and myriad other trinkets and goodies for sale on this lively street. This stretch of Abbot Kinney also offers numerous dining options. At the intersection of California Ave. are Abbot's Habit, a popular hangout offering deli sandwiches and a salad bar, and Tortilla Grill, an excellent and inexpensive "fresh Mex" eatery. Stroh's Gourmet sandwich and coffee shop sits a few short blocks farther down Abbot Kinney, just past Cadiz Ct.

- Just before you reach Westminster Ave., notice the low brick structure on the left with a faded metal sign that reads IRV'S FAMILY MARKET. The distinguished old building now houses art galleries.

- On the final block of Abbot Kinney, between Westminster and Main St., you'll see Lilly's, an elegant French restaurant, and restaurant-critic fave Joe's Restaurant on your right. The Westminster Ave. Elementary School is on your left.

- Turn left on Main St. This leg of the walk is a little drab compared to the thriving consumer mecca you've left behind on Abbot Kinney, but it does feature a few points of interest. As you approach the corner of Westminster Ave., you'll see the Westminster off-leash dog park on your right. This is a good place to stop if you've brought Fido along.

- Cross Westminster and continue on Main St. for about two blocks to the Windward Circle rotary, which was a picturesque lagoon back in Abbot Kinney's day, when more than 16 miles of canals snaked through "Venice of America."

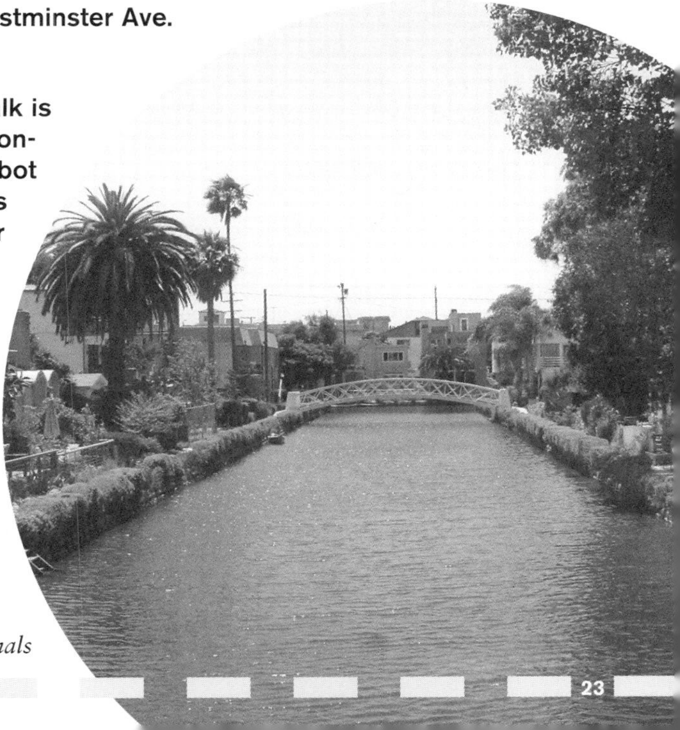

Venice canals

At this point, you may choose to turn right on Windward Ave., which will take you the few short blocks to the Venice Beach Boardwalk. Also known as Ocean Front Walk, this is a popular destination for tourists, inline skaters, and cyclists who like to cruise the waterfront. Sidewalk vendors hock incense, T-shirts, and various tourist-targeted wares of questionable value. If you do take this detour, return the way you came to the corner of Main St. and Windward.

- Walk along the west side of the rotary to remain on Main St.

- Turn left on Venice Way.

- Walk one block to Riviera Ave. and turn right. As Riviera crosses Mildred Ave., it becomes Dell Ave.

- Turn left immediately before the auto and pedestrian bridge, and follow the sidewalk alongside Carroll Canal.

- Continue straight along the sidewalk, pausing one last time to admire the unique and lovely homes on either side of the canal before crossing Eastern Ct. and returning to your starting point on Ocean Ave.

Back Story: Venice of America Amusement Park

The area now known as Venice was originally founded as "Venice of America" by real estate magnate Abbot Kinney in the fledgling years of the 20th century. This idealistic beach community was built on reclaimed marshland and featured an amusement park, a heated indoor saltwater "plunge," a miniature railroad, and more than 16 miles of canals, complete with Venetian gondolas and gondoliers. Unfortunately, expensive upkeep and the rise of the automobile meant that most of the canals were paved over by 1929, and the remaining six eventually fell into disrepair. Fortunately, those six were restored in the early '90s, and today the neighborhood built around the canals is affluent and idyllic. Come to think of it, it might have been more appropriate to name this sidebar "Backwater."

POINTS OF INTEREST

Venice Farmers Market Corner of Dell Ave. and South Venice Blvd., Venice, CA 90291, Fridays 7 A.M. to 11 A.M.

Abbot's Habit 1401 Abbot Kinney Blvd., Venice, CA 90291, 310-399-1171

Tortilla Grill 1357 Abbot Kinney Blvd., Venice, CA 90291, 310-581-9953

Stroh's Gourmet 1239 Abbot Kinney Blvd., Venice, CA 90291, 310-450-5119

Lilly's 1031 Abbot Kinney Blvd., Venice, CA 90291, 310-314-0004

Joe's Restaurant 1023 Abbot Kinney Blvd., Venice, CA 90291, 310-399-5811

Westminster Off-Leash Dog Park 1234 Pacific Ave., Venice, CA 90291, 310-301-1550

ROUTE SUMMARY

1. Head south on Ocean Ave.
2. Turn right on Linnie Ave.
3. Cross the bridge and immediately turn left to follow the sidewalk alongside Eastern Canal.
4. Follow the sidewalk as it turns right alongside Howland Canal.
5. Cross Dell Ave.
6. Turn right to follow the sidewalk alongside Grand Canal.
7. Cross the first bridge on the left and immediately turn right to follow the sidewalk on the other side of Grand Canal.
8. Follow the walkway up to South Venice Blvd. and turn right.
9. Turn left on Abbot Kinney Blvd.
10. Turn left on Main St.
11. Walk along the west side of the Windward Circle rotary to remain on Main St.
12. Turn left on Venice Way.
13. Turn right on Riviera St. Riviera turns into Dell Ave.
14. Turn left just before the bridge to follow the walkway alongside Carroll Canal.
15. Continue straight across Eastern Ct. and end back at Ocean Ave.

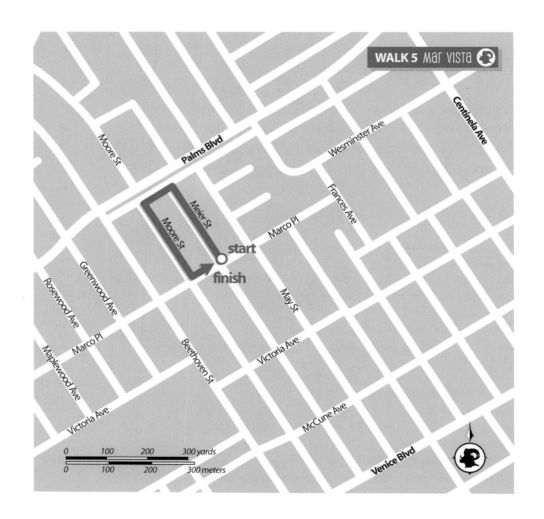

Moore St

Palms Blvd

Wesminster Ave

Centinela Ave

Meier St

Frances Ave

Moore St

Marco Pl

start

finish

Greenwood Ave

May St

Rosewood Ave

Marco Pl

Maplewood Ave

Beethoven St

Victoria Ave

Victoria Ave

McCune Ave

Venice Blvd

0   100   200   300 yards

0   100   200   300 meters

5 Mar Vista: a Utopian Vision of Modern Living

BOUNDARIES: Palms Blvd., Beethoven St., Venice Blvd., Centinela Ave.
THOMAS GUIDE COORDINATES: **Map 672; B4**
DISTANCE: **Approx. ¾ mile**
DIFFICULTY: **Easy**
PARKING: **Free street parking is available on Marco Pl.**

One of 1940s modernist architect Gregory Ain's finest achievements is a tract of houses in Mar Vista. This two-block housing project of 52 homes was marketed as the "Modernique Homes" when it was completed in 1948. The neighborhood embodies the now kitschy 1940s perception of progressive architecture; the one-story houses are modest in size and style, with low, flat roofs and high, rectangular windows. Nearly all of the structures in this neighborhood are uniform in design, but Ain gave each home its own look with carefully chosen interior and exterior color combinations. He also worked closely with Garrett Eckbo, a visionary of modern landscape design who created a rustic community landscape to further distinguish this zone from the surrounding neighborhood.

This very short walk explores Ain's successful handiwork; the Mar Vista tract remains, to this day, a peaceful, well-maintained collection of modest-sized homes in the rarefied air of Los Angeles' West Side. Some of these homes may even look vaguely familiar, as they've served as shooting locations for several modern-day television commercials.

● **Begin at the corner of Meier St. and Marco Pl. and head north, away from Marco Pl. The house on the northeast corner of Meier and Marco is a fine example of how Ain and Eckbo combined contemporary and rustic elements; the design of the home is unmistakably modern, but the unfinished wood-picket fence and thriving garden lend a country feel to the property.**

This harmonious juxtaposition is echoed all along Meier St., with its mature magnolia trees shading rows of homogenous houses, each with its own distinct color scheme and landscape design. The palette is muted: pale blues and greens, olive, and mustard—nothing so jarring as to interfere with the neighborhood's cohesiveness. You will notice some variance of design between the homes, however. For example, some

houses have overhanging roof extensions supported by diagonal stilts, while others have no such ornamentation to interfere with their boxy regularity. And the house at 3500 Meier is built on a slight incline at the end of the street, so it is a little larger than the rest, with the living space extended over a sunken garage.

- Turn left on Palms Blvd. While Palms is a fairly busy thoroughfare, this short portion of the street is separated from the main boulevard by a thickly landscaped meridian in order to shield the neighborhood from some of the traffic noise.

- Turn left on Moore St. Part of Eckbo's original vision for this neighborhood's landscape architecture was to give each street its own look with a particular species of tree, so while Meier got magnolias, Moore is trimmed with melaleucas, distinguished by their towering stature and peeling bark. The elegant home at 3501 Moore has polished wood trim and glass-brick windows. This is one of very few houses in the area that was not originally designed by Gregory Ain, although it does blend in nicely, with its low, flat roof and simple, rectangular shape. Across the street at 3508 is the original model house created by Ain, identified by the pink diagonal stilts supporting the roof extension above the front walkway.

DESIGNER NAME: GREGORY AIN

Gregory Ain was a second-generation modernist architect, influenced by first-wave modernists like Rudolph Schindler and Richard Neutra. In fact, one of Ain's greatest architectural influences was Schindler's Kings Road house in West Hollywood (see Walk 15). Ain's noble goal was to create a utopian residential life for people who couldn't afford large, ostentatious homes, so he designed stylish, dignified, and utilitarian apartments and houses for low- to middle-income families.

All of the houses in Ain's development are set close to one another, and there is a sense of communal living in the way the front yards flow into one another; very few homes along this street are separated by hedges or fences. The community landscaping is lush and shady, and the many varieties of palm trees give the neighborhood an almost tropical feel.

● Turn left on Marco Pl. to return to your starting point. Note that at the intersection with Marco Pl., both Moore St. and Meier St. are slightly offset from their continuation to the south, as if Gregory Ain's careful study in modern community living was purposefully set apart from its less carefully planned surroundings.

route summary

1. Begin at the intersection of Marco Pl. and Meier St. and head north on Meier St.
2. Turn left on Palms Blvd.
3. Turn left on Moore St.
4. Turn left on Marco Pl.

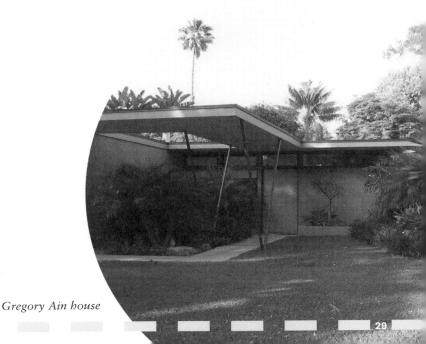

Gregory Ain house

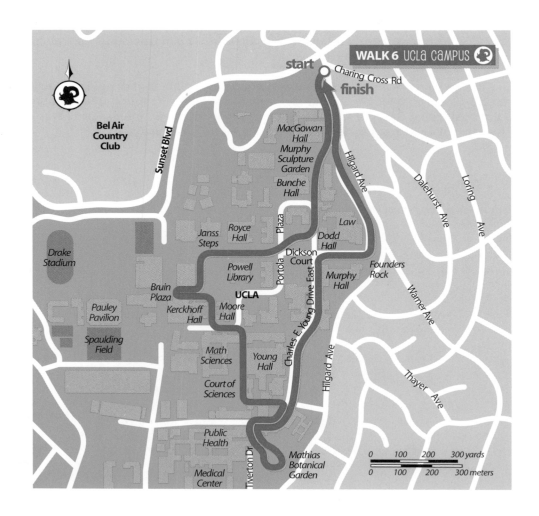

WALK 6 UCLA CAMPUS

start
finish
Charing Cross Rd

Bel Air
Country
Club

Sunset Blvd

Hilgard Ave

Dalehurst Ave

Loring Ave

MacGowan
Hall
Murphy
Sculpture
Garden

Bunche
Hall

Plaza

Law

Dodd
Hall

Janss
Steps

Royce
Hall

Drake
Stadium

Dickson
Court

Powell
Library

Portola

Murphy
Hall

Founders
Rock

Warner Ave

Bruin
Plaza

UCLA

Charles E. Young Drive East

Pauley
Pavilion

Kerckhoff
Hall

Moore
Hall

Spaulding
Field

Math
Sciences

Young
Hall

Hilgard Ave

Thayer Ave

Court of
Sciences

Public
Health

Tiverton Dr

Mathias
Botanical
Garden

0   100   200   300 yards

0   100   200   300 meters

Medical
Center

6 UCLA Campus:
Ivy League Style with a West Coast Twist

BOUNDARIES: **Sunset Blvd., Hilgard Ave., Le Conte Ave., Gayley Ave.**
THOMAS GUIDE COORDINATES: **Map 592; B1**
DISTANCE: **Approx. 1¾ miles**
DIFFICULTY: **Easy (includes stairways)**
PARKING: **Limited street parking is available on Hilgard Ave. south of Sunset Blvd. Paid parking is available on campus.**

UCLA is one of the most well-known campuses in the state's famed public University of California system. Renowned for its challenging academic programs as well as for its gorgeous, ideally situated campus, UCLA represents the mythical undergraduate experience that many of us wish we had had.

This route explores the most scenic spots on this massive campus, taking in innovative artwork, classically beautiful architecture, and a lovely botanical garden that has evolved over several decades.

● Begin on Hilgard Ave. just south of Sunset Blvd. Look for Charles E. Young Dr., which splits off from Hilgard to the right, and follow it south into the UCLA campus.

● Turn right at the semicircular driveway to head into the Franklin D. Murphy Sculpture Garden. Pass a shallow fountain on the right as you descend the short stairway into the sunken grassy area. Notice the two columns topped with bronze sculptures of nude dancers by Robert Graham. The sculpture garden spans more than 5 acres of UCLA's north campus and includes an eclectic blend of naturalistic and sleekly modern pieces from artists such as Alexander Calder, Henri Matisse, Jacques Lipchitz, and Auguste Rodin. It is the largest outdoor sculpture garden on the West Coast and one of the prettiest, with its rolling green lawns and feathery jacaranda trees. After taking some time to admire the sculptures and bas-reliefs (there are more than 70), return to the eastern end of the garden and follow the sidewalk south.

- As you head south along the sidewalk, on your right you'll come to Bunche Hall, which features an innovative indoor palm garden in its central atrium. Continue south along the sidewalk, passing Luvalle Commons on your left.

- When you reach Dodd Hall, turn right to follow the diagonal path through the sunken, shady lawn of Dickson Court, which is shaded by mature sycamore and fig trees.

- After crossing Portola Plaza, the street that borders Dickson Court, you'll find yourself in the university's Historic Quad. This wide-open, grassy area runs between the four original buildings of the Westwood campus, all of which were built in 1929 in the Italian Romanesque style. You'll pass Haines Hall on your right and Kinsey Hall on your left before coming to the campus's two most well-known landmarks. On your right is Royce Hall, which architect David Allison designed based on a basilica in Milan. Powell Library is on your left, and while it bears some architectural resemblance to Royce Hall, it was designed by another architect, George Kelham. Powell's octagonal tower and main entrance are modeled after two different churches in Italy. Part of what makes the northeast portion of the UCLA campus so beautiful is its architectural integrity; the red-brick, Italianate buildings lend a distinguished, Old World feel to the College of Humanities.

- Continue westward through the quad, and you'll come to the semicircular Royce Hall fountain on Janss Terrace. Descend the Janss Steps, which provided the original entrance to the university, leading up from Westwood Blvd. Admire the expansive view of the intramural fields stretched out in the distance. To your right is the Fowler Museum of Cultural History. The Student Activities Center lies on the south side of the lawn below, with Kaufman Hall sitting opposite. On this side of campus, the university's newer buildings, with their red-brick and tan-stone exteriors integrate beautifully with the original architecture.

- Turn left at the bottom of the stairs and follow the pathway heading south. Kerkhoff Hall lies straight ahead. Tree-shaded lawns roll gently alongside the sidewalk, yet another idyllic place for scholars to engage in or rest from their academic pursuits.

- At the end of the sidewalk, turn right to follow the Bruin Walk into Bruin Plaza, home of the Bruin Bear himself, a 2-ton bronze statue of a ferocious-looking grizzly. At the southeast corner of the plaza is Ackerman Union, a modern building distinguished by ship-like arched wood beams atop the roof. The UCLA store occupies the first floor of the building and offers just about anything a student would need to purchase, from groceries to designer apparel to Macintosh computers, as well as a diverse collection of dining options.

● Head back the way you came on Bruin Walk, past Ackerman Union, and return to Kerkhoff Hall. Built in 1931, this is the only building on campus with the Collegiate Gothic architectural style. Continue straight ahead up the steps, and then turn right (following the sign pointing toward the Kerkhoff Coffeehouse). Cross through the outdoor dining patio between Kerkhoff Hall and Moore Hall, which is on your left.

● Turn left on Portola Plaza; the Mathematical Sciences building is on your right. You are now entering into the more technical side of campus, which is not nearly as pretty as the Humanities section in terms of architecture.

● Just after you've passed the Math Sciences building, turn right to cross through the Court of Sciences. Boelter Hall is on your right; the Geology building, Young Hall, and Boyer Hall are on your left; and the newly constructed Life Sciences building is ahead.

● Just after passing Boyer Hall, turn left and follow the path back onto Charles E. Young Dr.

● Turn right on Young Dr. and follow it to the right, as it passes the curving brick façade of the newly constructed building on your right.

● Turn left on Tiverton Dr. You'll see the sign for the Mildred E. Mathias Botanical Garden on your left.

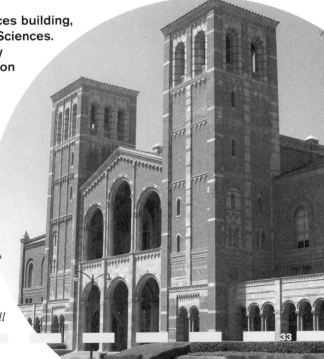

Royce Hall

- Follow the driveway entrance to the botanical gardens, just across the street from the School of Dentistry, and then enter the actual gardens through the North Gate on your right.

  Follow the gently sloping path that descends into the sunken gardens, and take the time to explore at your leisure, or perhaps simply sit and relax in the green shade on one of the many benches. This 7-acre oasis features plant life from all over the world, including many species of tropical and subtropical flora. The topography of UCLA's botanical gardens is a remnant of the ravine that used to run across the entire campus. Today, a water pump feeds the river that flows down the center of the gardens.

- After spending some time in the gardens, make your way back toward the point where you entered at the north end, and exit back out onto Tiverton Dr. Turn right on Tiverton.

- Turn right on Charles E. Young Dr. and continue along the perimeter of campus. After crossing Westholme, you'll notice the barn-like structure of the Faculty Center on your right.

- Just past Murphy Hall, turn right (instead of continuing straight, which would take you back to the sculpture garden) on a path that will take you past the School of Law on your left.

- Turn left to continue on Charles E. Young Dr., following it all the way back to the intersection with Hilgard Ave., where you began.

POINT OF INTEREST

Mildred E. Mathias Botanical Garden UCLA, Los Angeles, CA 90095, 310-825-1260.
Please call ahead to make sure the gardens are open at the time of your visit.

ROUTE SUMMARY

1. Begin on Hilgard Ave. just south of Sunset Blvd. and turn right on Charles E. Young Dr., which leads into the UCLA campus.
2. Turn right at the semicircular driveway to head into the Franklin D. Murphy Sculpture Garden.
3. Turn left to cut across the garden and continue straight along the sidewalk that heads south.
4. When you reach Dodd Hall, turn right to follow the diagonal path through Dickson Plaza.
5. Cross Portola Plaza to continue straight into UCLA's Historic Quad.
6. Cross the quad to the Janss Steps and descend.
7. Turn left at the bottom of the stairs and follow the pathway.
8. At the end of the sidewalk, turn right to follow the Bruin Walk into Bruin Plaza.
9. Head back the way you came on Bruin Walk. Continue straight ahead up the steps and then turn right. Cross through the patio between Kerkhoff Hall and Moore Hall.
10. Turn left on Portola Plaza; the Mathematical Sciences building is on your right.
11. Just after you've passed the Math Sciences building, turn right to cross through the Court of Sciences.
12. Just after passing Boyer Hall, turn left and follow the path back to Charles E. Young Dr.
13. Turn right on Young Dr. and follow it as it curves to the right.
14. Turn left on Tiverton Dr.
15. Follow the driveway entrance to the botanical garden on your left, and then enter through the North Gate on your right.
16. Exit the garden back out onto Tiverton Dr. and turn right.
17. Turn right on Charles E. Young Dr. and continue along the perimeter of campus.
18. Turn right on the path just past Murphy Hall.
19. Turn left to continue on Charles E. Young Dr., following it all the way back to your starting point at the intersection with Hilgard Ave.

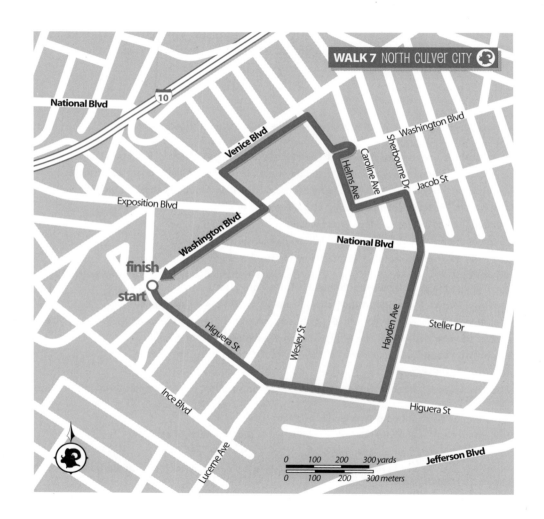

National Blvd

10

Venice Blvd

Exposition Blvd

Washington Blvd

Washington Blvd

Helms Ave

Caroline Ave

Sherbourne Dr

Jacob St

National Blvd

finish

start

Higuera St

Wesley St

Hayden Ave

Steller Dr

Ince Blvd

Luceme Ave

Higuera St

Jefferson Blvd

| 0 | 100 | 200 | 300 yards |
| 0 | 100 | 200 | 300 meters |

7 NOrTH CULVer CITY: HIDDEN Treasure ON THE WEST SIDE

BOUNDARIES: **Venice Blvd., Higuera St., Jefferson Blvd., La Cienega Blvd.**
THOMAS GUIDE COORDINATES: **Map 672; H1**
DISTANCE: **Approx. 1½ miles**
DIFFICULTY: **Easy**
PARKING: **Free street parking is available on Higuera St. Note: The Expo Line will include a stop near this route, but the first phase isn't planned for completion until 2010.**

Culver City is truly a gem on LA's West Side, and this route uncovers those characteristics that make it such a desirable place to live. Beginning in the picturesque neighborhood known as Rancho Higuera, this walk takes in some of the most innovative industrial-style architecture in all of Los Angeles, and then visits the trendy area around the historic Art Deco Helms Bakeries buildings, which are now home to chic eateries and upscale furniture stores.

● **Begin on Higuera St., just south of Washington Blvd. Head southwest on Higuera, away from Washington.** This is the main thoroughfare through the Rancho Higuera neighborhood, popular with commuters cutting between Washington and Jefferson boulevards. For this reason, residents had mini rotaries installed at each of the cross streets, which effectively slow down motorists. The homes on this street are modest in size and carefully maintained. Higuera is lined with flowering trees and bushes, with Baldwin Hills forming a pastoral backdrop to the southwest.

● **After several short blocks, turn left on Hayden Ave.** (Hayden Pl. heads into an office park to the right). You'll notice a brick building with a unique, stepped roofline on your left. This is the Debbie Allen (of *Fame* fame) Dance Academy, and it spans the length of a city block. Most of the buildings on this street are industrial warehouses, some of which are more worn down than others, yet it manages to retain the safe feel of the residential neighborhood you just left behind. At 3599 Hayden Ave., stop at J.J.'s Cafe, a decent little lunch spot marked with a green awning.

As you draw closer to National Blvd., you'll reach the Hayden Tract, an old industrial area now famed for its innovative architecture. On your left, at 3535, is a massive, free-form structure in light gray stucco, punctuated by sharp points and odd outcroppings. On the right is a collection of structures identified as "Conjunctive Points." The dominant building looks like something Darth Vader might call home. It looms over the street, all sharp angles in faded black metal and glass. The building on your right features a sort of brick bubble with three off-kilter windows that look as if they were tacked onto the otherwise featureless gray wall. This has got to be one of the most striking collections of buildings in LA.

- When you reach National Blvd., cross at the crosswalk and then continue straight on the sidewalk that passes through the oleander hedge on the other side of the railroad tracks.

- Continue straight ahead onto Sherbourne Dr., another shady residential street much like Higuera.

- Turn left on Jacob St. and continue across Caroline Ave.

- Turn right on Helms Ave. When you reach the corner of Helms Ave. and Washington Blvd., you'll leave the residential neighborhood behind. Cross Washington and then walk a few yards to your right to take a peek at the colorful public art piece depicting a Helms Bakeries truck crashing into a movie studio backdrop of Culver City. A knocked-over fire hydrant spurts water, completing the comical effect.

Continue north on Helms Ave. On your left is the sprawling Art Deco Helms Bakeries complex. Built in 1930 and then closed in 1969, the bakery warehouses have been kept in pristine condition and are now home to many businesses, mostly upscale furniture and antique stores. La Dijonaise, a top-notch French bakery and cafe, occupies the southeast corner of the building. In addition to fresh, tasty food, this eatery offers reasonable prices and a pleasant, airy atmosphere, making it a great place to stop for lunch, coffee, dessert, or all three. Next door to La Dijonaise is the Jazz Bakery, one of LA's premier spots to hear talented jazz and blues artists. And Beacon, a hip Asian eatery serving beautifully prepared and flavorful fusion cuisine ranging from pad thai to sashimi, is across the street on the east side of Helms Ave.

- Turn left on Venice Blvd. H.D. Buttercup, a huge, airy showroom where customers can purchase furnishings directly from more than 50 manufacturers, sits on the corner of Venice and Helms. This diverse and upscale furniture mart has received a great deal of buzz since opening in early 2005 and also features a restaurant, bar, and Helms Bakery Museum. Several more furniture stores line the south side of Venice Blvd.

- Turn left on National Blvd.

- Turn right on Washington Blvd. You'll notice the Jungle, a tropical plants nursery, on the northwest corner of National and Washington. The next couple of blocks are populated almost exclusively with new and used car dealers.

- Turn left on Higuera St. (the street is named Robertson Blvd. heading in the other direction) to return to your starting point. On your right is the neighborhood market, Jerry's Market Deli, on the corner of Poinsettia Ct., a quiet little alley of charming, closely set Spanish-style homes. This peaceful lane captures the spirit of Rancho Higuera, which is a pretty, safe, diverse, and utterly unpretentious neighborhood in a wonderfully central location.

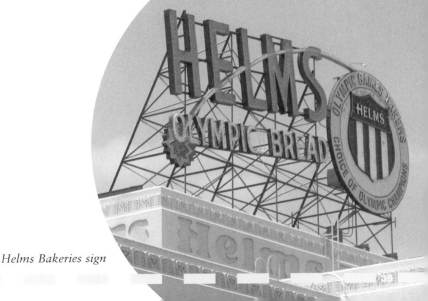

Helms Bakeries sign

POINTS OF INTErEST

J.J.'s Cafe 3599 Hayden Ave., Culver City, CA 90232, 310-837-3248
La Dijonaise 8703 Washington Blvd., Culver City, CA 90232, 310-287-2770
Jazz Bakery 3233 Helms Ave., Culver City, CA 90034, 310-271-9039
Beacon 3280 Helms Ave., Culver City, CA 90034, 310-838-7500
H.D. Buttercup 3225 Helms Ave., Culver City, CA 90034, 310-558-8900

route summary

1. Begin on Higuera St. just south of Washington Blvd. and head southwest on Higuera St.
2. Turn left on Hayden Ave.
3. Cross National Blvd. and continue straight through the pedestrian passageway onto Sherbourne Dr.
4. Head north on Sherbourne Dr.
5. Turn left on Jacob St.
6. Turn right on Helms Ave.
7. Turn left on Venice Blvd.
8. Turn left on National Blvd.
9. Turn right on Washington Blvd.
10. Turn left on Higuera St.

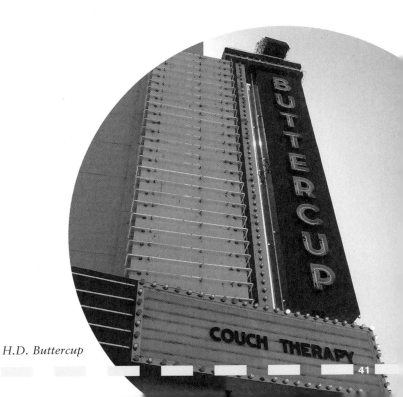

H.D. Buttercup

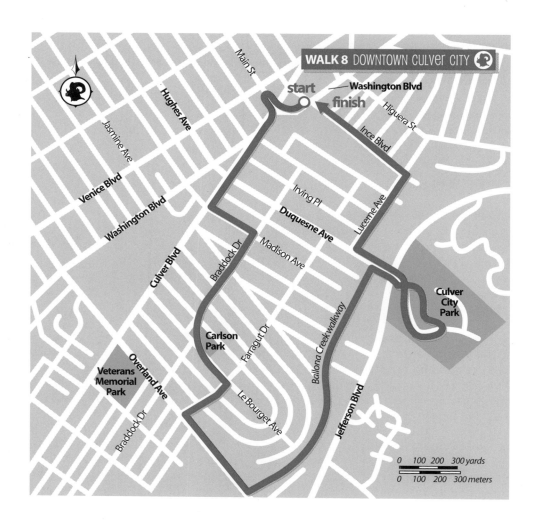

Main St

start

finish

Washington Blvd

Higuera St

Ince Blvd

Hughes Ave

Jasmine Ave

Venice Blvd

Washington Blvd

Irving Pl

Duquesne Ave

Lucerne Ave

Culver Blvd

Braddock Dr

Madison Ave

Carlson Park

Farragut Dr

Ballona Creek walkway

Culver City Park

Le Bourget Ave

Jefferson Blvd

Overland Ave

Veterans Memorial Park

Braddock Dr

0   100   200   300 yards

0   100   200   300 meters

8 DOWNTOWN CULVER CITY: HOLDING ONTO ITS PLACE IN MOVIE-MAKING HISTORY

BOUNDARIES: Venice Blvd., Overland Ave., Jefferson Blvd., Ince Blvd.
THOMAS GUIDE COORDINATES: Map 672; H1
DISTANCE: Approx. 3½ miles
DIFFICULTY: Moderate (includes stairways)
PARKING: Free street parking is available on Ince Blvd. Note: The Expo Line will include a stop near this route, but the first phase isn't planned for completion until 2010.

A quiet town on Los Angeles' otherwise high-profile West Side, Culver City is home to Sony Pictures Studios, as well as historic Culver Studios. It is said to have been a notorious spot for nightlife during Prohibition, and now downtown Culver City is enjoying a renaissance as an evening destination thanks to an influx of stylish and well-reviewed restaurants, as well as a thriving art gallery scene. The area also bustles with activity on weekdays, when purposeful young executives and interns from the studios run errands and power lunch at its broad selection of dining establishments.

● Begin at Culver Studios, on the corner of Ince Blvd. and Washington Blvd. The studio façade resembles a grand colonial mansion, which film buffs will instantly recognize from the opening credits of *Gone with the Wind*. Culver Studios was built by Thomas H. Ince in 1919, and has also been home to RKO, DeMille, and Desilu studios during its lifetime. Today it is owned by Sony Entertainment. Head northwest on Washington Blvd., away from Ince Blvd.

Immediately northwest of Culver Studios is the Culver Hotel, a six-story, triangular, brick building situated at the junction of Washington, Culver Blvd., and Main St. Another historic landmark, this establishment opened as the Hotel Hunt in 1924 to accommodate the many actors who filmed at the studios across the street. In fact, the "munchkins" from *The Wizard of Oz* had such a good time here that they held a reunion of the surviving cast members at the hotel in 1997. Take a few minutes to visit the hotel's elegant lobby, which has been restored with its original wood and marble.

- As long as you're here, you should head north to stroll up Culver City's one-block Main Street—locals like to brag that it's the shortest main drag in the United States. The Culver City Farmers Market sets up here every Tuesday from 3 P.M. to 7 P.M., later in the day than most of LA's farmers markets. BottleRock, a vibrant wine bar, is located at 3847 Main St. The street is also home to the Massage Garage, where you can get a one-hour massage for only $45; the Grand Casino Bakery, an Argentinean bakery and sandwich shop; Italian restaurant Novecento; La Ballona for Mexican food; a thrift shop; and an old-fashioned hardware store. The small-town feel of Culver City's diminutive Main St. contrasts sharply with the frantic commercial hubbub immediately to the north on Venice Blvd.

- Return to Culver Blvd. and turn right. Fraiche, a critically adored upscale restaurant serving French- and Italian-inspired cuisine, is located at 9411 Culver Blvd. This is one of several well-regarded eateries on this stretch; others include the Tender Greens gourmet salad bar at 9523 Culver and "gastropub" Ford's Filling Station at 9531. As if you didn't have enough tempting dining options to choose from, Santa Maria Barbecue is located at 9552 Washington Blvd., where Washington joins with Culver Blvd. Their tri-tip sandwich, served open-faced on garlic bread, is not to be missed. (If your mouth isn't watering yet, just wait until you catch a whiff of the smoky aroma coming from the restaurant.)

At the corner of Culver and Duquesne Ave. is City Hall, a collection of attractive Spanish-style, white-stucco buildings. Take a moment to wander under the freestanding arched entryway through the courtyard and admire the fountains.

Continue to head southwest on Culver, and you'll notice an imposing, stepped, granite-and-glass structure across the street on your right, at the intersection of Madison Ave. This is Sony Pictures Plaza. Directly opposite the entrance to the plaza on Madison is one of the gates to Sony Pictures Studios. You can't miss the signature water tower rising from the back lot. You can arrange a tour of the studios by calling 323-520-TOUR (there is a fee).

- Turn left on Madison Ave. to enter a quiet residential neighborhood of mostly modest houses. Culver City showcases an interesting assortment of architecture, and this neighborhood features everything from tidy bungalows to larger and, for the most part, uninspired, contemporary homes.

- Walk one block on Madison and then turn right on Braddock Dr. Continue for five short blocks to Dr. Paul Carlson Park.

- Cut diagonally southeast across the shady park to Le Bourget Ave. and turn left.

- Walk one block on Le Bourget and then turn right on Farragut Dr.

- After three quiet residential blocks, you arrive at busy Overland Ave., where you turn left.

- After about 0.3 mile, you'll come to the pedestrian entrance to the Ballona Creek walkway and bike path. Ballona Creek is a concrete-sided waterway that empties into the ocean in Marina del Rey, but today you will follow it inland. Take the pedestrian ramp down to the creek and continue to head northeast along the pathway. Depending on the time of year, there may be a sad little trickle or a healthy stream burbling through the channel.

- Follow the river walkway for just under a mile to Duquesne Ave. You can't miss the exit to the street, as it is marked by a whimsical metallic structure in the shape of a giant water urn, which stands next to the Culver City Transportation Center on the opposite side of the creek.

Culver Studios façade

- Turn right on Duquesne and walk to the intersection of Jefferson Blvd. Cross Jefferson and you're at the entrance to Culver City Park.

- Follow the road as it curves uphill, passing a playground on your right, and then turn left into the parking lot. This will take you to the base of a zigzagging wooden walkway that leads to the top of the hill. Once you reach the summit, take a few minutes to enjoy the panoramic view of West Los Angeles and the Pacific Ocean. Also take a second to check out the giant sundial sculpture, which proclaims itself an "Homage to Ballona Creek." The mosaic-tiled base of the sundial is decorated with the words "Time is a River" in several different languages.

- Turn right at the top of the ramp and walk around the perimeter of the baseball field. Descend the stairway behind the snack bar.

- Turn right on the service road at the bottom of the stairs and follow it to where it intersects with Duquesne. Continue down the hill on Duquesne to return to the intersection at Jefferson Blvd.

- Cross Jefferson and head northwest on Duquesne back in the direction of downtown Culver City.

- Turn right on Lucerne Ave., a quiet, tree-lined street that leads through another residential neighborhood.

- After about a third of a mile, you reach Ince Blvd. Turn left here. As you make your way down Ince, you'll notice a studio back lot on your left. This is the utilitarian lot that resides behind Culver Studios' ostentatious façade. On the right side of the street, at the intersection of Poinsettia, is a low, industrial-style building, cartoonishly ornamented with short orange columns. One column is intentionally crooked, giving the illusion that it is buckling under the weight of the roof. The name "Paramount Laundry Company" is engraved over the entrance.

- Return to your starting point at the intersection of Ince Blvd. and Washington Blvd.

POINTS OF INTEREST

Culver Hotel 9400 Culver Blvd., Culver City, CA 90232, 888-328-5837

Culver City Farmers Market Main St. between Culver Blvd. and Venice Blvd., Culver City, CA 90230, Tuesdays 3 P.M. to 7 P.M.

BottleRock 3847 Main St., Culver City, CA 90232, 310-836-9463

Massage Garage 3812 Main St., Culver City, CA 90232, 310-202-0082

Grand Casino Bakery 3826 Main St., Culver City, CA 90232, 310-202-6969

Novecento 3837 Main St., Culver City, CA 90232, 310-842-3838

La Ballona 3843 Main St., Culver City, CA 90232, 310-838-7409

Fraiche 9411 Culver Blvd., Culver City, CA 90232, 310-839-6800

Tender Greens 9523 Culver Blvd., Culver City, CA 90232, 310-842-8300

Ford's Filling Station 9531 Culver Blvd., Culver City, CA 90232, 310-202-1470

Santa Maria Barbecue 9739 Culver Blvd., Culver City, CA 90232, 310-842-8169

Sony Pictures Studios 10202 West Washington Blvd., Culver City, CA 90232, 323-520-TOUR

route summary

1. Begin on the corner of Ince Blvd. and Washington Blvd. and head northwest on Washington Blvd., away from Ince Blvd. to the intersection with Culver Blvd. and Main St.

2. Head north to stroll along one-block Main St.

3. Return to Culver Blvd. and turn right.

4. Turn left on Madison Ave.

5. Turn right on Braddock Dr.

6. Cut diagonally southeast across Dr. Paul Carlson Park to Le Bourget Ave. and turn left.

7. Turn right on Farragut Dr.

8. Turn left on Overland Ave.

9. Take the pedestrian entrance on your left down to the Ballona Creek walkway and bike path.

10. Follow the river walkway to Duquesne Ave.

11. Turn right on Duquesne and then cross Jefferson Blvd. to reach the entrance to Culver City Park.

12. Follow the road as it curves uphill, and then turn left into the parking lot and ascend the wooden walkway that leads up the hill from the parking lot.

13. Turn right at the top of the ramp and walk around the perimeter of the baseball field, and then descend the stairway behind the snack bar.

14. Turn right on the service road at the bottom of the stairs and follow it to where it intersects with Duquesne, and then continue down the hill to return to Jefferson Blvd.

15. Cross Jefferson and head north on Duquesne.

16. Turn right on Lucerne Ave.

17. Turn left on Ince Blvd. to return to your starting point.

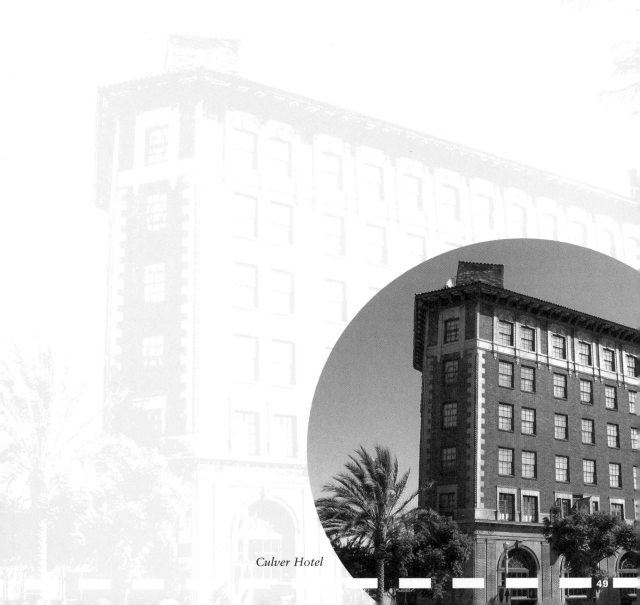

Culver Hotel

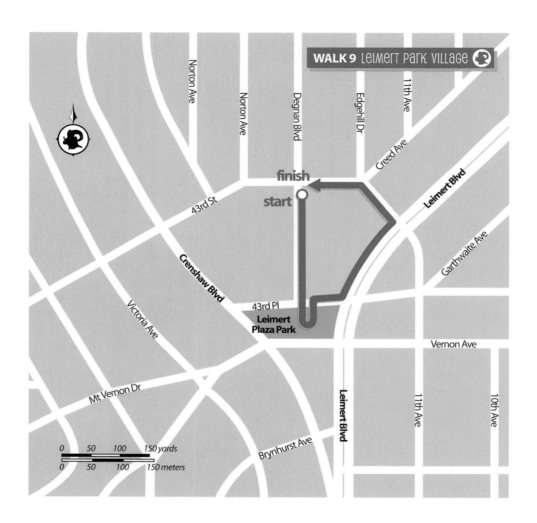

WALK 9 Leimert Park Village

Norton Ave

Norton Ave

Degnan Blvd

Edgehill Dr

11th Ave

Creed Ave

Leimert Blvd

Garthwaite Ave

43rd St

finish
start

Crenshaw Blvd

Victoria Ave

43rd Pl

Leimert
Plaza Park

Vernon Ave

Mt Vernon Dr

Leimert Blvd

11th Ave

10th Ave

Brynhurst Ave

0   50   100   150 yards
0   50   100   150 meters

9 Leimert Park Village: Preserving African-American Business and Culture

BOUNDARIES: **Crenshaw Blvd., 43rd St., Leimert Blvd.**
THOMAS GUIDE COORDINATES: **Map 673; F3**
DISTANCE: **Less than ½ mile**
DIFFICULTY: **Easy**
PARKING: **Metered parking is available on Degnan Blvd., south of 43rd St., and in a parking lot on the southeast corner. Free street parking is available on Degnan north of 43rd St.**

Leimert Park Village is truly a treasure in South Los Angeles. A revitalization effort that began more than 10 years ago has been dedicated to preserving this area for African-American small-business owners who place an emphasis on cultural enrichment. Due to the success of this movement, Leimert Park has become Los Angeles' main destination for Afrocentric dining, shopping, art, and entertainment, particularly dance, poetry, jazz, and blues. While the Village is a fine place to visit during the day, especially if you want to enjoy some authentic soul food or browse the shops for clothing, jewelry, and gifts, it really comes alive at night, when the sidewalks are crowded with enthusiastic patrons of the arts, and the air is saturated with the sounds of drum circles, jazz, blues, and passionate spoken-word performances.

● Begin at the intersection of 43rd St. and Degnan Blvd. To the north, Degnan is a shady residential street bordered by attractive, well-maintained duplexes. To the south, it is the bustling commercial focal point of Leimert Park Village. On the northeast corner, at 3351 W. 43rd St., is the Lucy Florence Coffee House/Le Florence Gallery, an architecturally innovative multiuse space that includes a cafe, art gallery, and theater. Twin brother proprietors Ron and Richard Harris named the establishment after their mother, and the company logo is a heartbreakingly lovely sepia reproduction of her solemn wedding photo. The Harris brothers are fierce advocates of multicultural creative arts, so they've opened their doors to all manner of performance art and art exhibitions. Stop in at Lucy Florence to grab a coffee or a cool drink and pick up some fliers about forthcoming shows and exhibitions—if you're lucky, you might even catch an interesting performance in progress.

A farmers market sets up in the Vision Theatre parking lot on the southeast corner of 43rd and Degnan every Saturday from 10 A.M. to 3 P.M. A colorful mural celebrating African-American musicians overlooks the lot.

- Head south on Degnan Blvd. At 4317, you'll come to M&M Soul Food Restaurant. This destination for authentic Southern-style cooking has expanded beyond South LA in recent years due to its popularity. A permanent sign declares this shop to be an "LAPD Stopping Location." This brings up an interesting fact about Leimert Park—though it's smack-dab in the middle of an area of Los Angeles that sees its fair share of crime, this enclave feels safe and vibrant, both day and night, as it has thrived as a positive community gathering place since its revitalization. Eso Won Books, specializing in African-American literature, is located at 4331 Degnan. (As of this writing, the independently owned bookstore is in danger of closing, much to the dismay of the community.) If you turn right into the alley just past the bookstore, you can view another vibrant mural painted on the south-facing wall. Entitled *The Last Stand: Unite*, the artwork depicts African anti-colonial leader Patrice Lumumba and groundbreaking jazz musician Eric Dolphy.

Across the street, at 4334 Degnan, is Zambezi Bazaar, an eclectic gift shop selling a vast selection of African jewelry and clothing, as well as African-American greeting cards, figurines, tapestries, and posters. You're likely to hear jazz, blues, or even spoken word drifting out of the World Stage Performance Gallery at 4344 Degnan, where the plain interior set up with folding chairs sums up the low-key vibe in the Village. If you like what you hear, grab a seat and enjoy the show (don't forget to drop a couple of bucks in the donation box).

- At the end of Degnan Blvd., cross 43rd Pl. to visit Leimert Plaza Park, a narrow greenway set around a circular fountain. Public restrooms are available in the park, and benches set underneath the trees make an excellent place to picnic or simply sit and relax.

- Cross back to the north side of 43rd Pl. and turn right, passing an old Art Deco building that now houses Sunny's Spot Coffee House, another place where you're likely to catch a live jazz performance, day or night.

- Turn left on Leimert Blvd. Babe's & Ricky's Inn, at 4339 Leimert Blvd., is one of LA's best venues for live blues music; the original location on Central Ave. opened in 1964 and played host to many a music legend. Continue for one block back to 43rd St.

- Turn left on 43rd St. Tantalizing, smoky aromas emanate from Phillip's BBQ, located on the southwest corner of Leimert Blvd. and 43rd St. Continue on 43rd St. around the corner. The Regency West Theatre, at 3339 43rd St., shares the same building as Lucy Florence—a large, pale green structure painted with the silhouettes of what appear to be ancient African warriors armed with spears. This supper club hosts all types of theatrical performances, but it is best known as a venue for urban poetry and comedy. Next, you'll come back to the Lucy Florence Coffee House and the starting point of your walk.

M&M Soul Food Restaurant

POINTS OF INTEREST

Lucy Florence Coffee House and Le Florence Gallery 3351 W. 43rd St., Los Angeles, CA 90008, 323-293-1356

Leimert Park Village Farmers Market Vision Theatre parking lot on the southeast corner of 43rd St. and Degnan Blvd., Los Angeles, CA 90008, Saturdays 10 A.M. to 3 P.M.

M&M Soul Food Restaurant 4317 Degnan Blvd., Los Angeles, CA 90008, 323-298-9898

Eso Won Books 4331 Degnan Blvd., Los Angeles, CA 90008, 323-290-1048

Zambezi Bazaar 4334 Degnan Blvd., Los Angeles, CA 90008, 323-299-6383

World Stage Performance Gallery 4344 Degnan Blvd., Los Angeles, CA 90008, 323-293-2451

Sunny's Spot Coffee House 3349 W 43rd Pl., Los Angeles, CA 90008, 323-291-4075

Babe's & Ricky's Inn 4339 Leimert Blvd., Los Angeles, CA 90008, 323-295-9112

Phillip's BBQ 4307 Leimert Blvd., Los Angeles, CA 90008, 323-292-7613

Regency West Theatre 3339 W. 43rd St., Los Angeles, CA 90008, 323-292-5143

route summary

1. Begin at the intersection of 43rd St. and Degnan Blvd.

2. Head south on Degnan Blvd.

3. At the end of Degnan Blvd., cross 43rd Pl. to visit Leimert Plaza Park.

4. Cross back to the north side of 43rd Pl. and turn right.

5. Turn left on Leimert Blvd.

6. Turn left on 43rd St. Continue around the corner on 43rd St. to return to your starting point at the intersection of Degnan Blvd.

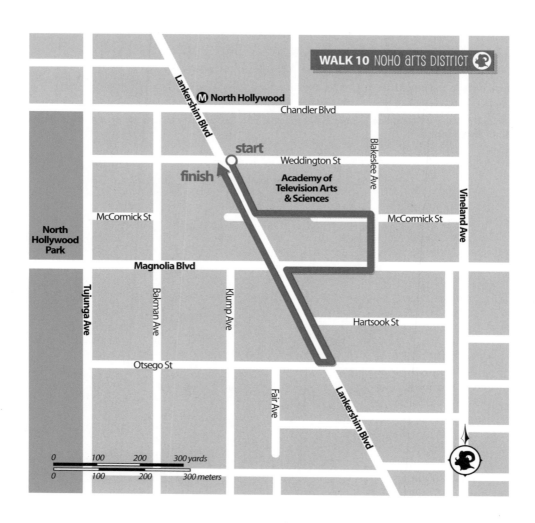

WALK 10 NOHO ARTS DISTRICT

Lankershim Blvd

M North Hollywood

Chandler Blvd

start

Weddington St

finish

Blakeslee Ave

Academy of
Television Arts
& Sciences

McCormick St

McCormick St

Vineland Ave

North
Hollywood
Park

Magnolia Blvd

Tujunga Ave

Bakman Ave

Klump Ave

Hartsook St

Otsego St

Fair Ave

Lankershim Blvd

| 0 | 100 | 200 | 300 yards |
| 0 | 100 | 200 | 300 meters |

10 NOHO ARTS DISTRICT: CREATIVITY BLOOMS IN THE MOST UNLIKELY PLACES

BOUNDARIES: **Chandler Blvd., Vineland Ave., Tujunga Ave., Otsego St.**
THOMAS GUIDE COORDINATES: **Map 562; J2**
DISTANCE: **Approx. ¾ mile**
DIFFICULTY: **Easy**
PARKING: **Metered parking is available on Lankershim Blvd.**
NEAREST METRO STATION: **Lankershim Blvd. and Chandler Blvd. (Red Line)**

North Hollywood's Lankershim Blvd. may hardly seem like a walking destination, but the birth of the NoHo Arts District makes it a neighborhood worth exploring. A stroll up and down the boulevard reveals a collection of art galleries, theater companies, and dance studios, as well as eclectic outdoor public art works that you wouldn't expect to encounter on this otherwise anonymous suburban thoroughfare deep in the San Fernando Valley.

- Begin at the northeast corner of Lankershim Blvd. and Weddington St. To the north, you'll see NoHo Commons, a high-rise housing development and shopping center that was built in 2007 to take advantage of the Metro Red Line station at Chandler Blvd. Head south on Lankershim.

- At 5220 Lankershim, you'll come to the Academy of Television Arts and Sciences complex. Enter the main plaza, passing the colorful whirligigs that adorn the lawn next to the driveway entrance. The plaza is surrounded by somewhat creepy-looking bronze busts of famous personalities such as Red Skelton, Bill Cosby, and Walt Disney, along with the unfamiliar faces of numerous company executives. The centerpiece is a massive, burnished statue of the Emmy award itself, which sits atop a circular tiered fountain.

- Exit the plaza via Blakeslee Ave., which heads south to Magnolia Blvd. Carefully cross Magnolia, a fairly busy street. The south side of Magnolia is home to several small theaters. The NoHo Arts Center, located at 11136, is devoted to multicultural performance art and theater. The vintage Avery Schreiber Theatre is located a few steps east of Blakeslee, at 11050 Magnolia. After picking up performance schedules at the theaters, head west on Magnolia back toward Lankershim.

● Turn left to head south on Lankershim. After passing the ubiquitous Starbucks on the corner, you'll come to the long black awning and big neon signs marking the entrance to the Eclectic Wine Bar & Grille, a neighborhood eatery that serves California cuisine and showcases the work of local artists.

● Cross Hartsook St. and continue south on Lankershim, passing under the giant retro sign for the North Hollywood Gym on the corner. You'll pass the Sanford Meisner Center, an acting school, at 5124, before coming to the cool, 1950s-style marquee for the Deaf West Theatre, at 5112. This theater company is a part of the Mark Taper Foundation that caters to deaf and hard-of-hearing performers and audiences throughout the country. The Lankershim Arts Center occupies a former Department of Water and Power office building with the DWP's trademark Art Deco exterior next door at 5108. The center is home to both the Road Theatre Company and NoHo Gallery LA.

● When you reach Otsego St., carefully cross Lankershim to head north back up the other side of the boulevard. The Citibank building on the southwest corner of Otsego and Lankershim catches the eye—a towering edifice of various geometric shapes, surface materials, and colors, it looks more like another art project than a financial institution. At 5113 Lankershim, you'll pass the Millennium Dance Complex, a dance studio that offers classes with professional choreographers.

Continue north on Lankershim. Pit Fire Pizza Company occupies an industrial-looking concrete building with an airy interior of exposed brick and corrugated metal on the northwest corner of Lankershim and Magnolia. A sign proclaims the pizza joint's mission of "Feeding a Hungry Nation." This is an excellent place to stop for a bite of mouth-watering, wood-fired pizzas with innovative toppings, or a delectable soup or sandwich. You can dine inside to enjoy the aroma of fresh-baked pizza crust, or outside to relax on the pleasant patio. Next door to Pit Fire is another public art display—a colorful mural depicting an idyllic park scene by artist Tim Fields.

Just north of Pit Fire, the collection of shops, galleries, and restaurants feature colorful neon and metal signs that compete for the attention of passers-by. The delightfully garish entrance to Tokyo Delve's Sushi Bar, at 5239, features squiggly neon letters and metal cutouts of classic Cadillacs. The kooky exterior design is an indicator of the crazy dining experience that awaits within—where diners are encouraged to dance on their chairs as everyone joins in on '80s sing-alongs.

The El Portal Theatre is located at 5269 Lankershim. Originally built in 1926 as vaudeville theater, the venue features a beautiful neon sign and gilded box office, and it is now home to three separate live performance theaters. The Bank Heist, a 1930s-themed restaurant and nightclub housed in a vintage brick bank building, sits on the northwest corner of Lankershim and Weddington.

● Cross Lankershim at Weddington to return to your starting point on the east side of the street.

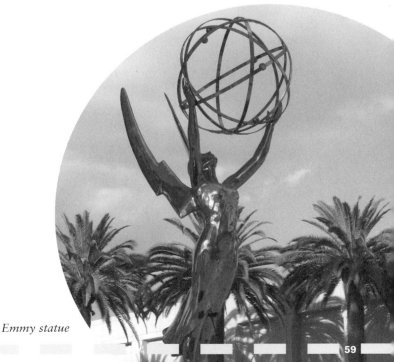

Emmy statue

POINTS OF INTEREST

Academy of Television Arts and Sciences 5220 Lankershim Blvd., North Hollywood, CA 91601, 818-754-2800

NoHo Arts Center 11136 Magnolia Blvd., North Hollywood, CA 91601, 866-811-4111

Avery Schreiber Theatre 11050 Magnolia Blvd., North Hollywood, CA 91601, 818-761-0704

Eclectic Wine Bar & Grille 5156 Lankershim Blvd., North Hollywood, CA 91601, 818-760-2233

Deaf West Theatre 5112 Lankershim Blvd., North Hollywood, CA 91601, 818-762-2998

Lankershim Arts Center 5108 Lankershim Blvd., North Hollywood, CA 91601, 818-760-1278

Pit Fire Pizza Company 5108 Lankershim Blvd., North Hollywood, CA 91601, 818-980-2949

Tokyo Delve's Sushi Bar 5239 Lankershim Blvd., North Hollywood, CA 91601, 818-766-3868

El Portal Theatre 5269 Lankershim Blvd., North Hollywood, CA 91601, 213-480-3232

Bank Heist 5303 Lankershim Blvd., North Hollywood, CA 91601, 818-760-1648

route summary

1. Begin at the corner of Lankershim Blvd. and Weddington St., and walk south on Lankershim.
2. Enter the Television Arts and Sciences plaza at 5220 Lankershim.
3. Exit the plaza via Blakeslee Ave., and turn right.
4. Turn right on Magnolia Blvd.
5. Turn left on Lankershim.
6. When you reach Otsego St., cross Lankershim to head north on the other side of the boulevard.
7. Cross Lankershim at Weddington to return to your starting point.

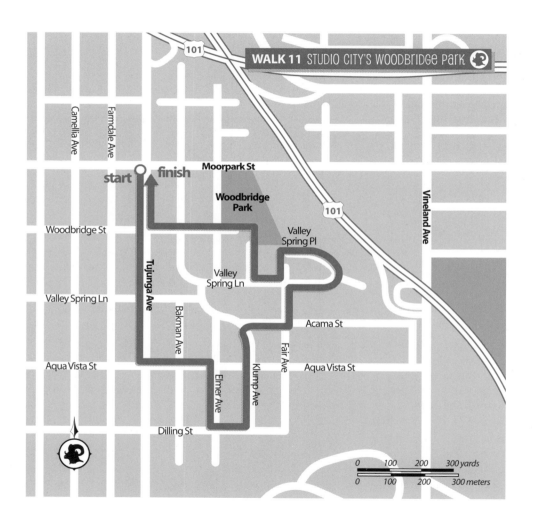

101

Camellia Ave

Farmdale Ave

Moorpark St

start **finish**

Woodbridge Park

101

Woodbridge St

Valley Spring Pl

Tujunga Ave

Valley Spring Ln

Valley Spring Ln

Bakman Ave

Vineland Ave

Acama St

Fair Ave

Aqua Vista St

Aqua Vista St

Elmer Ave

Klump Ave

Dilling St

0   100   200   300 yards

0   100   200   300 meters

11 STUDIO CITY'S WOODBRIDGE PARK: AN UNCANNILY FAMILIAR NEIGHBORHOOD

BOUNDARIES: **Moorpark St., Tujunga Ave., Ventura Blvd., Vineland Ave.**
THOMAS GUIDE COORDINATES: **Map 562; J4**
DISTANCE: **Approx. 1½ miles**
DIFFICULTY: **Easy**
PARKING: **Metered street parking is available on Tujunga Ave.**

Woodbridge Park is a preternaturally idyllic residential neighborhood in the Valley Village section of Studio City. The streets are shaded with mature trees and lined with meticulously maintained traditional homes. Bordered by the Los Angeles River on the south, the 101 Freeway on the northeast, and Tujunga Ave. on the west, this charismatic slice of affluent small-town America is effectively isolated from the anonymous sprawl of the surrounding Valley. Further, a neighborhood park and the collection of shops, salons, and restaurants in nearby Tujunga Village ensure that residents have little reason to leave their bucolic surroundings. It's no wonder why the Brady Bunch chose to settle down here.

● Begin at the corner of Tujunga Ave. and Moorpark St. and head south toward Woodbridge St. You are in the midst of Tujunga Village, a collection of neighborhood restaurants, shops, and salons that retains a distinctly small-town vibe. The Aroma Coffee and Tea Co., situated at 4360 Tujunga, is a big draw on this stretch; its ample patio seating makes it a great spot for dog owners, and the sandwiches, pastries, and coffee served by the friendly young staff are usually quite tasty. But for really good food, Caioti Pizza Cafe might be the better bet. Chef-owner Ed LaDou is famed for inventing California pizza (thin-crust pies with innovative toppings), but the restaurant is best known for its oddly named "The The Salad," a concoction of gorgonzola, balsamic vinegar, and walnuts said to induce labor in moms-to-be. Vitello's Italian Restaurant is located at 4349 Tujunga. This is the infamous spot where actor Robert Blake dined with his wife Bonnie Bakley just before she was found murdered in Blake's car, which was parked on a nearby side street. On a lighter note, Tujunga Village also features boutiques and salons, gourmet food stores, a yoga studio, Spoiled: A Day Spa, and the Two Roads Theatre.

- After you cross Woodbridge, Tujunga Ave. becomes a residential street lined with a mix of old and new apartment buildings. Tujunga is a main thoroughfare between Moorpark St. and Ventura Blvd., so traffic can be steady during rush hour.

- Turn left on Aqua Vista St., leaving the traffic of Tujunga behind as you enter an orderly suburban paradise of quiet, smoothly paved streets, carefully manicured lawns, and charming cottage-style homes. The dominant architectural styles are traditional ranch homes and wooden farmhouses, but Woodbridge Park also features a number of English cottages and Spanish-style homes.

- Turn right on Elmer Ave. You'll notice a colorful Southwest-style house on the southeast corner of Elmer and Aqua Vista. This vibrant home, sheltered by pine trees and innovatively adorned with abstract metal sculptures, stands out from the more traditional homes on this block. Continue to head south on Elmer Ave. Straight ahead, you can see the low, green hills of Studio City.

- Turn left on Dilling St. At 11222 Dilling is a familiar house—despite a new paint job and the addition of a low wall around the front yard, this home will be instantly recognizable by members of a certain generation as the Brady Bunch abode. Dilling is cut off from surrounding streets to the south and the east by the concrete-paved aqueduct that is somewhat misleadingly referred to as the Los Angeles River.

- Turn left to head north on Klump Ave., the street just opposite the Brady house. The ignobly named street is trimmed with eucalyptus, sycamore, and magnolia trees, whose ample shade provides welcome relief during hot Valley summers. A quaint stone cottage catches the eye at 4146 Klump. After crossing Aqua Vista, look for the owl statue perched atop the low, peaked roof of the garage at 4208 Klump.

- Turn right on Acama St. and continue for one block to Fair Ave. On the northeast corner of Fair and Acama is a home with a beautiful, abstract stained-glass window facing Acama.

- Turn left on Fair Ave. A very '60s-style apartment building resides at 4252 Fair, its colorful façade a jarring combination of stucco, wood, and stone.

- Turn right on Valley Spring Ln. At this point, the neighborhood starts to have a more rustic feel, as the sidewalks disappear and the foliage becomes a little overgrown. The rural vibe is somewhat spoiled by the noise of the adjacent 101 Freeway, however, as you continue to head east.

- Follow the road as it curves to the left, becoming Valley Spring Pl. When you reach the dead end, you'll see a low white fence on the left, constructed to prevent cars from trying to cut through the narrow passageway leading to Fair Ave. Cut through here, and continue to head south on Fair Ave.

- Turn right on Valley Spring Ln. and continue for one short block to Klump Ave.

- Turn right on Klump. At the end of the street, continue to head straight along the footpath that passes through a picket fence.

- The path emerges into the park for which this neighborhood is named. Woodbridge Park is a good-sized community-gathering place complete with a playground, recreation center, and jogging trails. Cut through the park, heading toward the southeast corner, where you will come upon the intersection of Elmer Ave. and Woodbridge St.

- Head west on Woodbridge, back toward Tujunga Ave. At the intersection of Bakman Ave., you'll see an English cottage that looks like it belongs in the pages of a children's storybook.

- Turn right on Tujunga Ave., returning to your starting point in Tujunga Village.

POINTS OF INTEREST

Aroma Coffee and Tea Co. 4360 Tujunga Ave., Studio City, CA 91604, 818-508-6505

Caioti Pizza Cafe 4346 Tujunga Ave., Studio City, CA 91604, 818-761-3588

Spoiled: A Day Spa 4338 Tujunga Ave., Studio City, CA 91604, 818-508-9772

Vitello's Italian Restaurant 4349 Tujunga Ave., Studio City, CA 91604, 818-769-0905

Two Roads Theatre 4348 Tujunga Ave., Studio City, CA 91604, 818-762-7488

route summary

1. Begin on Tujunga Ave. at Moorpark St. and head south on Tujunga.
2. Turn left on Aqua Vista St.
3. Turn right on Elmer Ave.
4. Turn left on Dilling St.
5. Turn left on Klump Ave.
6. Turn right on Acama St.
7. Turn left on Fair Ave.
8. Turn right on Valley Spring Ln.
9. Turn left on Valley Spring Pl.
10. Follow the pedestrian path on the left and then head south on Fair Ave.
11. Turn right on Valley Spring Ln.
12. Turn right on Klump Ave. and follow the pedestrian path into Woodbridge Park.
13. Cut across to southwest corner of Woodbridge Park.
14. Head west on Woodbridge St.
15. Turn right on Tujunga Ave.

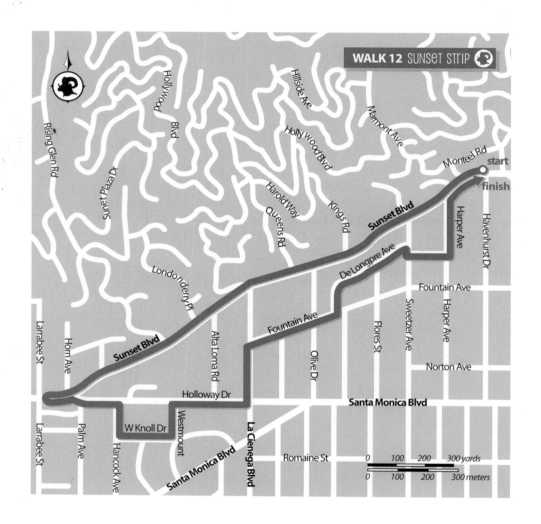

Rising Glen Rd

Hollywood Blvd

Hillside Ave

Marmont Ave

Hollywood Blvd

Montcel Rd

start

finish

Sunset Plaza Dr

Harold Way

Kings Rd

Sunset Blvd

Queens Rd

Harper Ave

Havenhurst Dr

De Longpre Ave

Londonderry Pl

Fountain Ave

Fountain Ave

Sweetzer Ave

Harper Ave

Sunset Blvd

Alta Loma Rd

Olive Dr

Flores St

Norton Ave

Larrabee St

Horn Ave

Holloway Dr

Santa Monica Blvd

W Knoll Dr

Westmount

La Cienega Blvd

Larrabee St

Palm Ave

Hancock Ave

Santa Monica Blvd

Romaine St

| 0 | 100 | 200 | 300 yards |
| 0 | 100 | 200 | 300 meters |

12 SUNSET STRIP: WHERE THE BEAUTIFUL PEOPLE COME TO PLAY

BOUNDARIES: Sunset Blvd., Crescent Heights Blvd., San Vicente Blvd., Santa Monica Blvd.
THOMAS GUIDE COORDINATES: Map 593; A5
DISTANCE: Approx. 2½ miles
DIFFICULTY: Easy
PARKING: Free street parking is available on Havenhurst Dr. before 6 P.M. Metered parking is available on Sunset Blvd.

West Hollywood's Sunset Strip is considered a tribute to Hollywood's colorful history by some, a den of iniquity to others, and a horrific traffic jam for east-west commuters. One thing's for sure, you can't drive along this stretch of Sunset Blvd. without being distracted by provocative billboards, giant, flashing video screens, and an endless stream of very attractive people, either dining on restaurant patios or, in some cases, shooting a scene for a movie. All this adds up to a fender bender waiting to happen, so better to park the car and walk a portion of this glitzy stretch of road so often identified with the City of Angels. This route also affords a peek at some of West Hollywood's architecturally significant apartment buildings that lie below the Strip and off the neon path.

● Begin at the intersection of Havenhurst Dr. and Sunset Blvd. On the northwest corner, mysteriously shrouded behind dense foliage, is the notorious Chateau Marmont. We've all heard the stories of John Belushi's overdose and the Jim Morrison's leap from a balcony, but the seven-story white castle and its tight-lipped staff continue to play impeccable hosts to a steady parade of present-day Hollywood A-listers and their indecorous shenanigans.

Head west on Sunset—your attention is caught by endless billboards and a string of partying/dining establishments, like trendy Japanese restaurant Miyagi's at 8225, and the Cabo Cantina, a funky outdoor margarita and taco joint at 8301. Speaking of indecorous behavior, the Body Shop strip club sits on the southwest corner of Sunset and Harper Ave.

- Cross Sweetzer Ave., and you'll come to the relentlessly hip Standard Hotel (note the quirky upside-down sign). Take a minute to wander through the retro, space-age-themed lobby outside to the poolside bar, which affords a spectacular view of the city below.

- Head back out to the street and continue west, passing Carney's Restaurant (housed in a train car) at 8351. The Saddle Ranch Chop House also sits on the north side of the street—notice the disheveled-looking mannequins of Old West characters leaning out over the balconies. It gets even rowdier inside, where a mechanical bull completes the *Urban Cowboy* scene. Soon you'll come to the loveliest structure on Sunset—the Sunset Tower Hotel. This Art Deco landmark opened its doors as the Sunset Tower apartments in 1929, and past residents include John Wayne, Bugsy Siegel, and Howard Hughes.

  As you approach Olive Dr., you'll come to the ramshackle, Deep South-themed shanty that is the House of Blues. Bankrolled by one of the original Blues Brothers, Dan Aykroyd (along with John Belushi's brother Jim), this high-profile but relatively intimate venue gives concertgoers the chance to get up close and personal with their favorite musicians. If you're so inclined, drop into the Porch Restaurant upstairs for some stick-to-your-ribs soul food. The Comedy Store is directly across the street.

- Continue west on Sunset across La Cienega Blvd. You're now approaching Sunset Plaza, a short stretch of the boulevard devoted almost entirely to expensive shops and restaurants. This is a great area for celebrity spotting, and also a popular destination for foreign tourists with a lot of disposable income who are looking for the mythical "LA" experience. You'll pass Armani Exchange, BCBG, and many smaller clothing boutiques and shoe stores, as well as several upscale eateries like Caffe Primo, Cafe Med, and Il Sole, which feature prominent patio seating where patrons are sure to be seen. A few affordable eating options are available as well, such as Mel's Drive-In and Poquito Mas.

- When you reach the intersection of Sunset, Holloway Dr., and Horn Ave., continue straight ahead about a half block to Book Soup, an independent bookstore and newsstand worth checking out. This cozy shop is known for celebrity book signings. You'll notice a striking five-story silver building directly across the street; this is media conglomerate IAC/InterActiveCorp's West Coast headquarters, designed by superstar architect Frank Gehry.

- After browsing Book Soup's crowded aisles, retrace your steps to the intersection of Sunset and Holloway and continue straight ahead to remain on Holloway.

- Turn right on Hancock Ave. and follow it for one block to W. Knoll Dr.

- Turn left on W. Knoll Dr., a pleasantly quiet and shady residential street.

- At the intersection with Westmount Dr. is a small traffic rotary graced with a lovely tiled pillar and flowering plants. Turn left to head uphill on Westmount.

- Turn right to get back onto Holloway Dr. and continue to La Cienega Blvd.

- Cross La Cienega and turn left on La Cienega to head back uphill toward Sunset Blvd.

- One block before Sunset, turn right on Fountain Ave. On the north side of the street is "the Villas," a beautiful courtyard apartment building built in the early 1930s. This is part of West Hollywood's Courtyard Thematic District, designed to preserve some of the region's architecturally significant multifamily housing from the 1920s and '30s.

- Turn left on De Longpre Ave. and follow the road as it curves to the right, passing behind the Sunset Tower Hotel before you come to William S. Hart Park on your left.

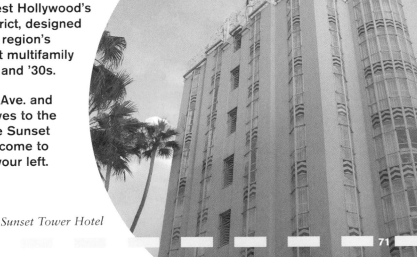

Sunset Tower Hotel

- Follow the path up to this popular gathering spot for neighborhood residents, which includes an off-leash dog park, an AIDS memorial garden, and the quaint, shingled house that has long been the West Coast headquarters of the Actors Studio. Descend the stairs back down to De Longpre and continue east.

- When the street ends, turn right on Sweetzer Ave., and then take an immediate left to get back on De Longpre.

- Turn left on Harper Ave. You are now in the Harper Ave. District, featuring more period revival apartment complexes built during the 1920s and '30s. Several gorgeous Spanish-style apartment buildings line the east side of the street. Casa Real, at 1354 Harper, is particularly interesting, with its muted tile work and copper fixtures that have turned a lovely slate-green with age. The 7 Fountains, at 1414, features a sculpture of an angel overlooking the front steps and is prettily embellished with colorful tile work.

- Turn right on Sunset Blvd., retracing your steps to your starting point at the corner of Havenhurst.

POINTS OF INTEREST

Chateau Marmont 8221 W. Sunset Blvd., West Hollywood, CA 90046, 323-656-1010

Miyagi's 8225 W. Sunset Blvd., West Hollywood, CA 90046, 323-650-3524

Cabo Cantina 8301 W. Sunset Blvd., West Hollywood, CA 90069, 323-822-7820

Standard Hotel 8300 W. Sunset Blvd., West Hollywood, CA 90069, 323-650-9090

Carney's Restaurant 8351 W. Sunset Blvd., West Hollywood, CA 90069, 323-654-8300

Saddle Ranch Chop House 8371 W. Sunset Blvd., West Hollywood, CA 90069, 323-656-2007

Sunset Tower Hotel 8358 W. Sunset Blvd., West Hollywood, CA 90069, 323-654-7100

House of Blues/Porch Restaurant 8430 W. Sunset Blvd., West Hollywood, CA 90069, 323-848-5100

Comedy Store 8433 W. Sunset Blvd., West Hollywood, CA 90069, 323-656-6225

Poquito Mas 8555 W. Sunset Blvd., West Hollywood, CA 90069, 310-652-7008

Mel's Drive-In 8585 W. Sunset Blvd., West Hollywood, CA 90069, 310-854-7200

Caffe Primo 8590 W. Sunset Blvd., West Hollywood, CA 90069, 310-289-8895

Cafe Med 8615 W. Sunset Blvd., West Hollywood, CA 90069, 310-652-0445

Il Sole 8741 W. Sunset Blvd., West Hollywood, CA 90069, 310-657-1182

Book Soup 8818 W. Sunset Blvd., West Hollywood, CA 90069, 310-659-3110

William S. Hart Park 8341 De Longpre Ave., West Hollywood, CA 90069, 323-848-6308

route summary

1. Begin at the intersection of Havenhurst Dr. and Sunset Blvd. and head west on Sunset.
2. When you reach the intersection of Sunset, Holloway Dr., and Horn Ave., continue straight ahead about half a block to Book Soup.
3. Retrace your steps to the intersection of Sunset and Holloway and continue straight ahead to remain on Holloway.
4. Turn right on Hancock Ave.
5. Turn left on W. Knoll Dr.
6. Turn left on Westmount Dr.
7. Turn right to get back onto Holloway and continue for one more block to La Cienega Blvd.
8. Cross La Cienega and turn left to head back uphill toward Sunset Blvd.
9. Turn right on Fountain Ave.
10. Turn left on De Longpre Ave. and follow the road as it curves to the right.
11. Follow the path up into Hart Park and then head down the stairs back to De Longpre and continue east.
12. Turn right on Sweetzer Ave., and then take an immediate left to get back on De Longpre.
13. Turn left on Harper Ave.
14. Turn right on Sunset Blvd., retracing your steps to Havenhurst.

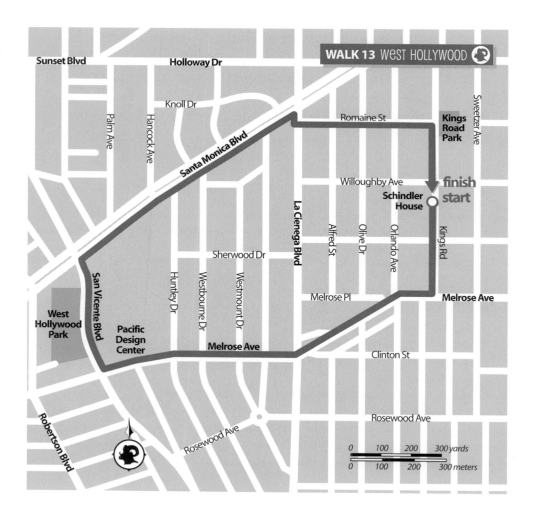

Sunset Blvd

Holloway Dr

Knoll Dr

Palm Ave

Hancock Ave

Santa Monica Blvd

Romaine St

Kings Road Park

Sweetzer Ave

Willoughby Ave

finish start

Schindler House

La Cienega Blvd

Alfred St

Olive Dr

Orlando Ave

Kings Rd

Sherwood Dr

San Vicente Blvd

Huntley Dr

Westbourne Dr

Westmount Dr

Melrose Pl

Melrose Ave

West Hollywood Park

Pacific Design Center

Melrose Ave

Clinton St

Robertson Blvd

Rosewood Ave

Rosewood Ave

| 0 | 100 | 200 | 300 yards |
| 0 | 100 | 200 | 300 meters |

13 WEST HOLLYWOOD: a STUDY IN INTERIOR AND EXTERIOR DESIGN

BOUNDARIES: Melrose Ave., San Vicente Blvd., Santa Monica Blvd., Kings Rd.
THOMAS GUIDE COORDINATES: Map 593; A6
DISTANCE: Approx. 2 miles
DIFFICULTY: Easy
PARKING: Free street parking is available on Kings Rd.

This tour of the best West Hollywood has to offer begins at the Schindler House, an early modern architectural gem and home of LA's MAK Center for Art and Architecture. The walk then goes on to explore the *tres chic* stretch of Melrose Ave. that is home to countless home furnishing galleries and antique stores, as well as Eastern-influenced establishments like Dr. Tea's Tea Garden & Herbal Emporium and the Bodhi Tree Bookstore.

Easily the most dramatic destination on this journey is the Pacific Design Center, a colossal structure of blue and green glass colloquially known as the "Blue Whale" that houses over a hundred interior design showrooms. From there, you'll pass through the commercial center of West Hollywood along Santa Monica Blvd. before returning to your starting point on Kings Rd.

● Begin on Kings Rd., just south of Willoughby Ave. The Schindler House sits at 835 Kings Rd., hidden from view by a tall bamboo hedge. Proceed along the dirt path to the MAK Center office and bookstore, where you can submit a donation before exploring the building. The Schindler House is a building like no other. Composed of unadorned concrete and dark-stained wood, the one-story building manages to feel airy and light despite the low, wood-beamed ceilings. Furnishings are modern and sparse, and a couple of rooms feature copper-topped fireplaces. The indoor and outdoor space is seamlessly integrated; clear plastic curtains separate the rooms of the house from the peaceful green gardens, which are shrouded from the surrounding area by more bamboo.

- After leaving the Schindler House, continue south on Kings Rd. toward Melrose Ave. Next door to the Schindler House is a new apartment complex called Habitat 825. The sleek, neo-modern structure was designed by Lorcan O'Herlihy and has received some flack for the way it towers over the south side of Schindler's famed creation, although the architect did made an effort to respect his neighbor when designing the building.

- Turn right on Melrose. Across the street is the Mel & Rose Wine Store, which is graced by a delightfully tacky giant wine bottle with a neon sign. Sweet Lady Jane is located at 8360 Melrose Ave. This family-owned dessert shop and bakery offers a staggering array of sweets (including gorgeous, mouthwatering special-occasion cakes) that have been written up in everything from *Zagat* to *W* magazine.

- Keep to the left at the fork in the road to avoid wandering onto Melrose Pl., which is home to a cache of snooty designer boutiques such as Marc Jacobs, Marni, and Carolina Herrera (unless, of course, you're in the mood for a very pricey shopping spree). Continue along Melrose Ave. Both sides of the street are lined with an interesting collection of furniture stores, antique shops, and galleries.

DESIGNER NAME: RUDOLF M. SCHINDLER

Rudolf M. Schindler was an Austrian-born architect who was inspired by Frank Lloyd Wright. After he began working for Wright in Chicago in 1918, his mentor sent him to Los Angeles to supervise the construction of the Hollyhock House (see Walk 23). It was here that Schindler established himself as an innovative and progressive architect in his own right. In 1922, he created West Hollywood's Kings Road House (now commonly referred to as the Schindler House), a building that is considered an icon of early modern architecture. Built in the early 1920s, the minimalist structure is an example of what Rudolf M. Schindler described as "space architecture." It functioned as his home and studio until he died in 1953. The space communicates a singular blend of old and new; while the building design is undoubtedly modern, the low ceilings and organic, unadorned materials reveal the influence of indigenous architecture.

● Cross La Cienega Blvd. At this point, you can see the Pacific Design Center looming ahead, and it's obvious why it came to be known as the "Blue Whale." On the southwest corner of La Cienega and Melrose is a singularly ugly strip mall composed of black and white, horizontally striped marble.

After crossing Westmount Dr., you'll find yourself in West Hollywood's ultra-hip enclave of Far East influence. At 8565 Melrose is Urth Caffe, an ostensibly healthy eatery that is invariably crowded with beautiful people looking to indulge in rich foods made with guilt-free ingredients. Next door, at 8585, is the Bodhi Tree Bookstore, which sells incense, candles, and other spiritual paraphernalia in addition to new and used books on topics ranging from Zen Buddhism to women's health. Across the street, at 8612, is Dr. Tea's Tea Garden & Herbal Emporium, which sells an array of proprietary herbal beverages. Behind the teahouse is a large botanical garden that provides a serene respite for patrons, with its trickling central fountain and comfy wicker chairs. Dr. Tea's also has a licensed herbalist and tarot card reader on site, as well as bodywork services (reflexology and acupuncture) and various classes, including tai chi and yoga.

At 8687 Melrose Ave., just before San Vicente Blvd., you finally arrive at the Pacific Design Center. Up close, the massive blue glass structure is striking—and almost intimidating. At night, the effect is even more dramatic, as the tall, pod-shaped spotlights bathe the building's exterior in a red glow. The Design Center is home to 130 showrooms displaying furniture and interior design pieces from an array of designers and manufacturers, ranging in style from traditional to contemporary. The center also frequently hosts exhibitions, lectures,

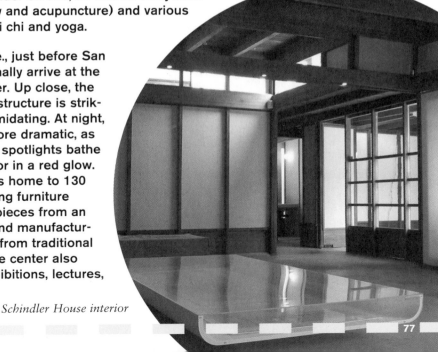

Schindler House interior

and special events. The Museum of Contemporary Art (MOCA) even has a satellite gallery here.

- The main entrance to Pacific Design Center is located around the corner on San Vicente. You'll pass a giant metal sculpture of a chair as you turn the corner. The entryway is situated off of a large, open courtyard, which is dominated by a spectacular dancing fountain. Call ahead or visit www.pacificdesigncenter.com to see if there is an exhibit worth seeing either at MOCA or in the Design Center at the time of your visit. Across the street, at 647 N. San Vicente, you'll notice West Hollywood Park, which features a public swimming pool and tennis courts.

- After exploring the Design Center, continue north on San Vicente, passing the sheriff's station on your right at the corner of Santa Monica Blvd.

- Turn right on Santa Monica. You are now in the heart of gay West Hollywood, as evidenced by the rainbow flags and names like LA Buns, Rage, and Trunks on the stores, bars, and restaurants along this stretch. To the north, you can spot the hotels and oversized billboards of the Sunset Strip.

- Continue east along Santa Monica for just under three quarters of a mile. This section is populated with a multitude of coffeehouses, juice bars, and frozen yogurt shops. Santa Monica Blvd. also reflects West Hollywood's residents' profound sense of self-improvement, with its collection of gyms, Pilates and yoga studios, UV-free tanning salons, and health stores.

The original Pinkberry location sits just south of Santa Monica on Huntley Dr. This insanely popular fro-yo shop serves an unusually tart (and purportedly healthy) frozen treat and has spawned dozens of new stores throughout the Los Angeles area (along with countless imitators). Innovative convenience store Famima!! is located a short distance northeast of Pinkberry, at 8525 Santa Monica Blvd. The stylish stop is a good place to grab a bite, as it features a delectable array of panini, sushi, noodle dishes, pastries, and various Eastern-flavored snacks.

- When you reach La Cienega Blvd., turn right and then take an immediate left on Romaine St. You have now left the hustle and bustle of the boulevard and entered a quiet residential neighborhood. The shady street is lined with the ubiquitous Spanish-style apartments and houses, as well as a few Norman-style cottages.

- After four blocks, Romaine St. ends at Kings Road Park, a delightful, dog-friendly haven tucked between two apartment buildings. The shady little park features benches arranged around a burbling fountain, a small playground, and public restrooms, as well as dog waste bags to ensure that owners clean up after their pooches.

- After visiting the park, head south on Kings Rd. toward your starting point. The street is lined with courtyard apartment buildings; a narrow, dark-shingled complex at 906 N. Kings Rd., the "Tree House," stands out from the rest.

- Cross Willoughby Ave. to return to your starting point near the Schindler House, at 835 Kings Rd.

POINTS OF INTEREST

Schindler House and MAK Center for Art and Architecture 835 N. Kings Rd., West Hollywood, CA 90069, 323-651-1510

Sweet Lady Jane 8360 Melrose Ave., West Hollywood, CA 90069, 323-653-7145

Urth Caffe 8565 Melrose Ave., West Hollywood, CA 90069, 310-659-0628

Bodhi Tree Bookstore 8585 Melrose Ave., West Hollywood, CA 90069, 310-659-1733

Dr. Tea's Tea Garden & Herbal Emporium 8612 Melrose Ave., West Hollywood, CA 90069, 310-657-9300

Pacific Design Center and MOCA 8687 Melrose Ave., West Hollywood, CA 90069, 310-657-0800

Pinkberry 868 Huntley Dr., West Hollywood, CA 90069, 310-659-8285

Famima!! 8525 Santa Monica Blvd., West Hollywood, CA 90069, 310-659-2684

route summary

1. Begin at the Schindler House at 835 Kings Rd., just south of Willoughby Ave.
2. Head south on Kings Rd.
3. Turn right on Melrose Ave.
4. Keep left on Melrose Ave. to avoid Melrose Pl.
5. Turn right on San Vicente Blvd. to reach the entrance of the Pacific Design Center.
6. Turn right on Santa Monica Blvd.
7. Turn right on La Cienega Blvd. and then take an immediate left on Romaine St.
8. At the end of Romaine St., enter Kings Road Park.
9. Exit the park and head south on Kings Rd.
10. Cross Willoughby Ave. to reach starting point at 835 Kings Rd.

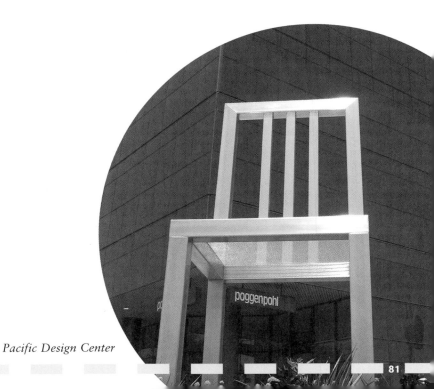

Pacific Design Center

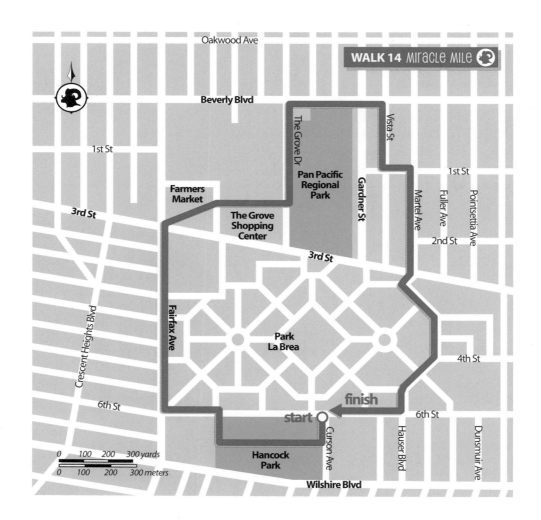

Oakwood Ave

Beverly Blvd

1st St

3rd St

The Grove Dr

Pan Pacific
Regional
Park

Vista St

Gardner St

Martel Ave

Fuller Ave

Pointsettia Ave

1st St

2nd St

Farmers
Market

The Grove
Shopping
Center

3rd St

Crescent Heights Blvd

Fairfax Ave

Park
La Brea

4th St

6th St

6th St

finish

start

Curson Ave

Hauser Blvd

Dunsmuir Ave

Hancock
Park

Wilshire Blvd

0   100   200   300 yards
0   100   200   300 meters

14 miracle mile: 40,000 years in the making

BOUNDARIES: Wilshire Blvd., Fairfax Ave., Beverly Blvd., Martel Ave./Hauser Blvd.
THOMAS GUIDE COORDINATES: Map 633: C2
DISTANCE: Approx. 2½ miles
DIFFICULTY: Easy
PARKING: Free parking is available on the north side of 6th St. Metered parking is available on the south side.

The Miracle Mile district is a prized area in Los Angeles, in large part due to its proximity to just about anyplace you might want to go. This neighborhood is home to the Los Angeles County Museum of Art (LACMA), the historic Farmers Market, and—unlikely as it may seem in the middle of this bustling city—one of the world's most famous fossil sites. The La Brea Tar Pits, located adjacent to LACMA, is said to have the largest and most diverse collection of animal and plant fossils from the last ice age, tens of thousands of years ago. After exploring the tar pits and fossil excavation sites, you'll get a strong dose of modern-day Los Angeles at The Grove, an enormously popular outdoor mall created by mega-developer Rick Caruso that brings to mind Disneyland's Main Street USA.

● **Begin at the corner of 6th St. and Curson Ave. and head south on Curson (toward Wilshire Blvd.).**

● **Just before you reach Wilshire, you'll see an entrance to Hancock Park on your right. This park is home to the tar pits and the Page Museum, which oversees the preservation, study, excavation, and cleaning of fossils from the tar pits. The Los Angeles County Museum of Art is also here.**

● **Enter Hancock Park (there are public restrooms near the entrance) and notice the Page Museum on your right. Take a few minutes to follow the steps to the roof of the building, and you'll be rewarded with a view over the museum's lush tropical garden and koi pond. It's peaceful up here, with the sound of a trickling waterfall and birds flitting in and out of the oasis below. The garden is topped with an intricate, open ironwork cage of sorts, the sides of which are decorated with a bas-relief of prehistoric creatures.**

- Return to ground level and walk south across the park to observe the largest of the tar pits, where the smell of liquid asphalt is reminiscent of hot days on the playground. The Page Museum has erected a heartbreaking sculptural tableau of a baby mammoth accompanied, presumably, by its father on the shore of the pond; the baby is wailing in sadness as it watches its mother get sucked into the muck. You can still see evidence of geologic activity on these grounds, with the occasional bubbling up of gases through the water's murky surface.

- Head west through the park, away from Curson. Hancock Park is a popular place for locals to walk their dogs, play Frisbee, or simply stroll across the hilly green lawns. You'll pass the Pavilion for Japanese Art on your left; this building, with its swooping architectural style, is part of LACMA. Continue through the park, passing a fossil excavation site on your right and the LACMA complex on your left. Soon, you reach the entry pavilion for the Broad Contemporary Art Museum building. This boxy travertine structure was designed by Renzo Piano and opened in 2008.

- Turn right opposite the entry pavilion to exit the park.

- Turn left on 6th St.

Back Story: Rancho La Brea Tar Pits

The Page Museum located at the site of Rancho La Brea gives visitors a taste of Los Angeles as it was 10,000 to 40,000 years ago, during the final Ice Age of the Pleistocene Epoch. The source of the asphalt pits that serve as the museum's excavation sites is a large underground petroleum reservoir located a short distance north of the park.

This extraordinarily sticky piece of land was the site of roughly 10,000 creatures' demise over the span of 30,000 years. The unlucky victims included small and large mammals, birds, and insects (but no dinosaurs, which were long since extinct during the Pleistocene Epoch). After an animal, such as a saber-toothed cat or dire wolf, became stuck in the goo, it would fall prey to carnivorous mammals and birds, some of which would themselves get caught in the mire. Today, the resulting collection of Ice Age fossils is one of the largest and most diverse in the world.

- Walk one block to Fairfax Ave., turn right, and continue for about half a mi... western side of the massive Park La Brea apartment complex occupies several blocks on your right. On your left, you'll pass Molly Malone's Irish Pub, at 575 Fairfax. Mani's Bakery, a health food cafe and bakery specializing in all-natural, wholesome desserts (which are actually quite tasty, if a bit dry at times) sits at 519 Fairfax. And you won't miss the four-story Art Deco building that's home to Samy's Camera at 431 Fairfax.

- Cross 3rd St. and enter the Farmers Market right next to the sign that reads MEET ME AT THIRD AND FAIRFAX.

- Walk into the market through the entrance near DuPar's restaurant, and make your way through the maze of food stands, coffee shops, butchers, bakeries, produce counters, and souvenir shops at this popular spot. Needless to say, this is a great place to grab a bite. Notable eateries include Loteria, a Mexico City-style taco stand, the Gumbo Pot for Cajun food, Pampas Grill Brazilian Churrascaria, the Banana Leaf for Singaporean food, and the French Crepe Company. As you make your way through the market, head toward the northeast corner, where you will exit straight into The Grove shopping center.

- Finding your way through The Grove is easy, as it's pretty much laid out in a straight line. It might not be so easy to make it through without blowing your paycheck, however. Most of the stores here are upscale, with an emphasis on men's and women's clothing. There are also several nice restaurants, a huge movie theatre, an Apple computer store, and a Barnes and Noble.

Rancho La Brea Tar Pits

The Grove distinguishes itself from Southern California's other outdoor malls with an old-fashioned trolley (a rather silly attraction, as this shopping center is less than a half mile long) and a large fountain shooting streams of water that "dance" to the tunes of old standards by crooners like Dean Martin and Frank Sinatra. It all makes for quite a spectacle, and it draws people in droves.

- After passing the Gap, turn left to exit the mall through the valet parking area onto The Grove Dr. and turn left.

- On your right is Pan Pacific Regional Park. This sunken expanse of rolling green lawns, playgrounds, playing fields, and jogging paths is relatively hidden from view of the surrounding streets, making it a delightful discovery if you're new to the area. Take some time to explore the park, which is usually filled with picnicking families and young athletes.

- Continue north on The Grove Dr. to the corner of Beverly Blvd. On the southwest corner is Erewhon Natural Foods Market. This oddly named store (it *almost* spells "nowhere" backward) is the destination for any sort of vegetarian, vegan, organic, Kosher, macrobiotic, herbal, or gluten-free delicacy you could desire. The market also features a juice bar and an extensive prepared foods counter that shopkeepers refer to as a "healthy-catessan." If you've managed to hold out this long without stopping at one of the many eateries on this walk, you may want to pick up a wrap or sandwich to take on a picnic in the park across the street.

- Turn right on Beverly Blvd., passing the post office on the south side of the street before you come to the Pan Pacific Park Recreation Center, which is constructed of red- and green-painted bricks. Its curvy outer wall lends the structure a pleasing, organic quality. Across the street, at 7619–21 Beverly Blvd., is Brooks Massage Therapy, an affordable, back-to-basics massage center with a natural-rock and eucalyptus steam room and no-nonsense massage therapists.

- Turn right on Vista St. to enter the Historic Preservation Overlay Zone (HPOZ), known as Miracle Mile North. (An HPOZ is an area that the city of Los Angeles has determined to have historic, architectural, aesthetic, or cultural significance.) Continue along Vista for one block, taking note of the various residential architectural styles.

The modest-sized homes are beautifully maintained, their preservation carefully over-seen by the HPOZ board. The predominant styles are Spanish Colonial Revival, Tudor Revival, and American Colonial Revival.

- Turn left on 1st St., and take note of the striking Norman cottage on the southeast corner.

- After one short block, turn right on Martel Ave. Here you'll spot a classic example of the American Colonial Revival architectural style on the southeast corner, at 100 S. Martel. Continue south on Martel. After you cross 2nd St., notice the collection of distinctive Spanish duplexes on your right, from 187 to 217 S. Martel. The congruity of layout and the intricate wrought-iron details suggest that these buildings were all designed by the same talented architect.

- Cross 3rd St. At this point, Martel Ave. becomes Hauser Blvd. Continue on Hauser for several blocks through the Park La Brea apartment complex. On your left, look for the relatively new, Italian-influenced Palazzo division of the complex. On your right are the original Park La Brea high-rises, which more closely resemble an inner-city housing project than a high-priced apartment complex.

- Turn right on 6th St. and then cross Curson to return to the start of your walk.

POINTS OF INTEREST

Page Museum 5801 Wilshire Blvd., Los Angeles, CA 90036, 323-934-7243

Los Angeles County Museum of Art 5905 Wilshire Blvd., Los Angeles, CA 90036, 323-857-6000

Mani's Bakery 519 S. Fairfax Ave., Los Angeles, CA 90036, 323-938-8800

Farmers Market 6333 W. 3rd St., Los Angeles 90036, 323-933-9211

The Grove 189 The Grove Dr., Los Angeles, CA 90036, 888-315-8883

Pan Pacific Regional Park 7600 Beverly Blvd., Los Angeles, CA 90036, 323-939-8874

Erewhon Natural Foods Market 7660 Beverly Blvd., Los Angeles, CA 90036, 323-937-0777

Brooks Massage Therapy 7619-21 Beverly Blvd., Los Angeles, CA 90036, 323-937-8781

route summary

1. Begin at the corner of 6th St. and Curson Ave. and head south on Curson.
2. Enter Hancock Park on your right to explore the Page Museum.
3. Visit the main tar pits on the south side of the park, opposite the Page Museum.
4. Head west through Hancock Park.
5. Exit the park by turning right opposite the entry pavilion for the Broad Contemporary Art Museum building.
6. Turn left on 6th St.
7. Turn right on Fairfax Ave.
8. Cross 3rd St. and enter the Farmers Market, heading toward the northeast corner.
9. Exit the Farmers Market and enter The Grove shopping complex.
10. Exit The Grove by turning left on The Grove Dr.
11. Turn right on Beverly Blvd.
12. Turn right on Vista St.
13. Turn left on 1st St.
14. Turn right on Martel Ave.
15. Cross 3rd St., where Martel Ave. becomes Hauser Blvd.
16. Turn right on 6th St. and then cross Curson Ave. to return to your starting point.

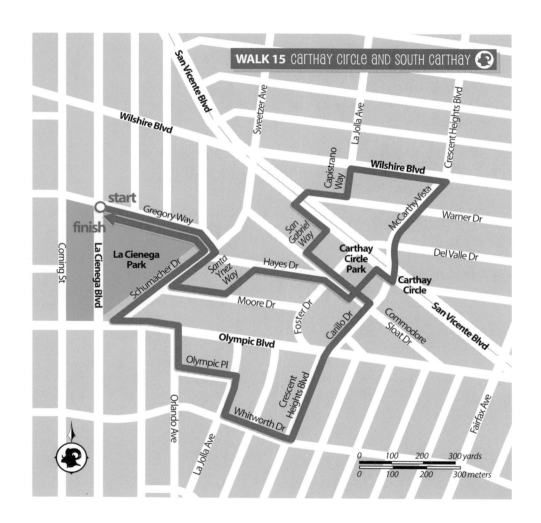

San Vicente Blvd

Sweetzer Ave

La Jolla Ave

Crescent Heights Blvd

Wilshire Blvd

Capistrano Way

Wilshire Blvd

McCarthy Vista

Warner Dr

start

Gregory Way

finish

Coming St

La Cienega Blvd

La Cienega Park

San Gabriel Way

Del Valle Dr

Carthay Circle Park

Santa Ynez Way

Hayes Dr

Schumacher Dr

Carthay Circle

Moore Dr

Foster Dr

Carillo Dr

San Vicente Blvd

Commodore Sloat Dr

Olympic Blvd

Olympic Pl

Orlando Ave

Crescent Heights Blvd

Fairfax Ave

La Jolla Ave

Whitworth Dr

0   100   200   300 yards

0   100   200   300 meters

15 Carthay circle and south carthay: an oasis of domestic harmony

BOUNDARIES: La Cienega Blvd., Wilshire Blvd., Fairfax Ave., Whitworth Dr.
THOMAS GUIDE COORDINATES: Map 632; J2
DISTANCE: Approx. 2 miles
DIFFICULTY: Easy
PARKING: Metered parking is available on La Cienega Blvd. and Gregory Way.

This walk explores the neighborhoods of Carthay Circle and South Carthay in Los Angeles' bustling Miracle Mile district, just southeast of Beverly Hills. Although they are right next to each other, these two neighborhoods—whose houses and apartment buildings have distinct architectural integrity and cohesiveness—have been designated as separate Historic Preservation Overlay Zones by the city of Los Angeles. Carthay Circle is primarily composed of Spanish Colonial Revival-style homes, with a few Tudor Revival and American Colonial Revival houses. The homes of South Carthay are a little more cohesive, consisting almost entirely of Spanish Colonial Revival structures. Both neighborhoods are well maintained and relatively isolated from the busy surrounding boulevards, making this a peaceful respite in the middle of one of LA's thriving business districts.

- The first part of this walk covers Carthay Circle, which features a mix of single-family homes and duplexes in an appealing variety of architectural styles, ranging from Spanish Colonial Revival to Tudor. Begin at La Cienega Park, situated on the east side of La Cienega Blvd. at the corner of Gregory Way. Head east on Gregory along the northern border of the park.

- Turn right on Schumacher Dr. At 865 Schumacher is an interesting stone house with parapets atop the roof that give it the incongruous look of a medieval castle.

- Turn left on Moore Dr. Notice the pair of Spanish-style homes on the northeast and southeast corners, each of which is dominated by a squat, tower-like structure.

- After less than a block, turn left on Santa Ynez Way, a narrow, slightly overgrown sidewalk alley.

- Santa Ynez emerges onto Hayes Dr. Turn right here.

- Hayes Dr. boasts an interesting variety of homes. At 6518 Hayes is a shingle-covered residence that echoes the Cape Cod architectural style. A low-lying brick house is located at 6513, and at 6444 Hayes is a lovely Spanish Colonial Revival home, distinguished by three perfect arches above the front patio and driveway.

- At the three-way intersection of Hayes, Commodore Sloat Dr., and Foster Dr., bear right onto Commodore Sloat.

- After about a half block, you'll see Carthay Circle Park—a narrow greenway between two office buildings—on your left. Turn left to cut through the park to San Vicente Blvd. At the end of the park, facing San Vicente, notice the sculpture of Juan Bautista de Anza, who led the first settlers from Sonora, Mexico, to California.

- Turn right on San Vicente, cross Carrillo Dr., and then take the crosswalk across San Vicente.

BACK STORY: MIRACLE MILE'S AUSPICIOUS BEGINNING

The conceit of the Miracle Mile district is that there doesn't appear to be anything miraculous about it. It's a vibrant and pleasant neighborhood, to be sure, with its distinctive mix of cultural institutions, tall office buildings, and charming residential neighborhoods. But it doesn't appear to be any grander than LA's other affluent districts.

The stretch of Wilshire Blvd. between La Brea Ave. and Fairfax Ave. was dubbed "Miracle Mile" when developer A.W. Ross decided to transform the dusty, 18-acre expanse of land into a prestigious shopping and business district in the 1920s. To this day, many of the original commercial buildings along Wilshire bustle with corporate activity, a dream come true for Ross. His original designation stuck, and the surrounding area has come to be known as the Miracle Mile district.

- Continue straight on the street that is now called McCarthy Vista for two short blocks to Wilshire Blvd.

- On the southeast corner of Wilshire Blvd. and McCarthy Vista is Wahoo's Fish Taco, a popular eatery with fresh food, quick service, and reasonable prices. Originally founded in San Diego, Wahoo's locations now dot Los Angeles County.

- After noshing on a taco or two, turn left to head west on Wilshire.

- At La Jolla Ave., you'll see an alley cutting between two tall office buildings on your left—turn here. This drab alley turns into Capistrano Way, a peaceful sidewalk trimmed with bougainvillea.

- As you emerge from Capistrano Way, you're faced with a remarkably lovely, yellow, Spanish-style home at 6354 Warner Dr. Turn right on Warner.

- Warner ends at San Vicente Blvd. Carefully cross San Vicente (a grassy island dividing this busy street makes jaywalking easy, but not necessarily legal).

- Once across San Vicente, you'll see a sign for San Gabriel Way a short distance to the southeast (to your left); this is yet another charming sidewalk alley. Turn right to follow San Gabriel Way through to Commodore Sloat Dr. Notice the striking American Colonial Revival house opposite the alley at 6440 Commodore Sloat.

- Turn left on Commodore Sloat and walk about two blocks.

- Turn right on Carrillo Dr. Carthay Circle Elementary School is on your right.

- When you reach the intersection with Olympic Blvd., cross the street using either the crosswalk or the underground tunnel (thoughtfully built for the safety of the schoolchildren).

- Now you are in the neighborhood of South Carthay. Continue straight on what is now Crescent Heights Blvd. This block is distinguished by gorgeous, immaculately maintained, Spanish-style duplexes and small apartment buildings.

- Turn right on Whitworth Dr. and continue for two blocks to La Jolla Ave.

- Turn right on La Jolla. Here, the residences are primarily one-story, single-family homes. The predominant architectural style is Spanish Colonial Revival, identified by its low-pitched, red-tile roofs and arched doorways and windows. Notice that many of these Spanish Colonial houses feature stained-glass details in the windows, just one example of the many decorative accents that distinguish this timelessly elegant architectural style. It is obvious why the city of Los Angeles chose to designate this as a protected architectural district.

- Turn left on Olympic Pl. and continue for one block to Orlando Ave.

- Turn right on Orlando and walk one block to Olympic Blvd.

- Turn left on Olympic. On the south side of Olympic, you'll notice several apartment buildings in the chateau-like French Normandy architectural style, which stand out from the other residences in the area.

- Turn right on Schumacher Dr. and continue for two blocks to Gregory Way.

- Turn left on Gregory Way to return to your starting point. At this point, you may need to use the facilities, which are conveniently located in nearby La Cienega Park.

POINTS OF INTEREST

La Cienega Park Community Center 8400 Gregory Way, Beverly Hills, CA 90211, 310-550-4625

Wahoo's Fish Taco 6258 Wilshire Blvd., Los Angeles, CA 90048, 323-933-2480

route summary

1. Begin at the corner of La Cienega Blvd. and Gregory Way and head east on Gregory.
2. Turn right on Schumacher Dr.
3. Turn left on Moore Dr.
4. Turn left on Santa Ynez Way.
5. Turn right on Hayes Dr.
6. Bear right onto Commodore Sloat Dr.
7. Turn left to cut through Carthay Circle Park.
8. Turn right on San Vicente Blvd., cross Carrillo Dr. to reach crosswalk, and then cross San Vicente Blvd.
9. Continue straight on McCarthy Vista.
10. Turn left on Wilshire Blvd.
11. Turn left into the alley opposite La Jolla Ave. This becomes Capistrano Way.
12. Turn right on Warner Dr.
13. Cross San Vicente Blvd. and head southeast (to your left) for a short distance to San Gabriel Way.
14. Turn right to pass through the San Gabriel Way alley.
15. Turn left on Commodore Sloat Dr.
16. Turn right on Carrillo Dr.
17. Cross Olympic Blvd.
18. Continue straight on Crescent Heights Blvd.
19. Turn right on Whitworth Dr.
20. Turn right on La Jolla Ave.
21. Turn left on Olympic Pl.
22. Turn right on Orlando Ave.
23. Turn left on Olympic Blvd.
24. Turn right on Schumacher Dr.
25. Turn left on Gregory Way.

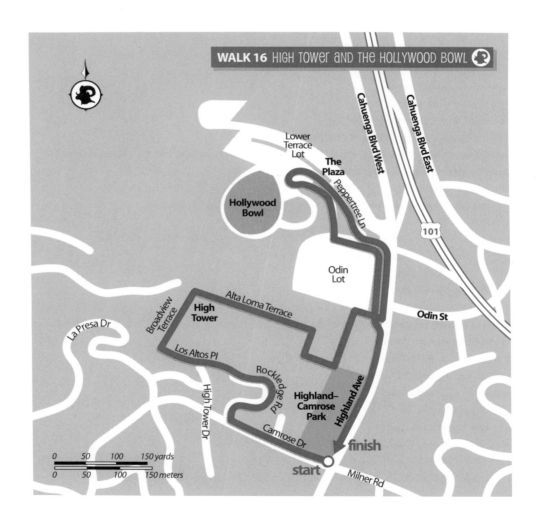

Lower
Terrace
Lot

The
Plaza

Cahuenga Blvd West

Cahuenga Blvd East

Peppertree Ln

Hollywood
Bowl

101

Odin
Lot

Odin St

Alta Loma Terrace

Broadview Terrace

High
Tower

La Presa Dr

Los Altos Pl

Rockledge Rd

Highland–
Camrose
Park

Highland Ave

High Tower Dr

Camrose Dr

finish

start

Milner Rd

0   50   100   150 yards
0   50   100   150 meters

16 HIGH TOWER AND THE HOLLYWOOD BOWL: HIDEAWAY IN THE HILLS

BOUNDARIES: **Highland Ave., Camrose Dr., 101 Freeway**
THOMAS GUIDE COORDINATES: **Map 593; E3**
DISTANCE: **Approx. 1 mile**
DIFFICULTY: **Moderate (includes stairways)**
PARKING: **Free street parking is available on Camrose Dr. Please be aware that parking anywhere in this vicinity on summer evenings can be problematic due to Hollywood Bowl parking restrictions.**
NEAREST METRO STATION: **Hollywood Blvd. and Highland Ave. (Red Line)**

Hollywood is bordered to the north by hills that provide a haven for those residents who crave privacy and quiet but still wish to remain close to the action. The neighborhood that lies adjacent to the Hollywood Bowl is one such retreat—a cozy, peaceful collection of homes, many of which are accessible only by stairway or by the "High Tower," an elevator tower for which the area is known. This excursion provides a rare glimpse into the hidden sanctuary sometimes referred to as Hollywood Heights.

- **Begin at the northwest corner of Highland Ave. and Camrose Dr. at Highland-Camrose Park. If the park's corner entrance is unlocked, you can enter here; otherwise, use the main entryway on Camrose Dr. This sanctuary is walled off from busy Highland Ave. to provide a convenient picnic area for patrons of the Hollywood Bowl, which lies just to the north. It's an interesting spot; in addition to rows of picnic tables and shaded lawns, the park features several Los Angeles Philharmonic Orchestra offices housed in colorful little bungalows, as well as a small police station. Public restrooms are also available here.**

- **Walk northwest through the park and exit through the main gateway onto Camrose. Turn right, passing a retirement home and several apartment buildings on your left, and cute, single-family bungalows on your right.**

- Turn right on Rockledge Rd. The cottage-style house on the northeast corner of Camrose and Rockledge boasts a meticulously tended rose garden out front. Straight ahead, look for the gorgeous, white stucco, Spanish-style home with extensive blue tile work and a long balcony of arches overlooking the front courtyard.

- Follow the road as it curves uphill. The Mediterranean houses are increasingly ornate and colorful as you continue up, and some even have castle-like architectural flourishes.

- At the cul-de-sac, you reach Los Altos Pl., a pedestrian walkway. Descend the short flight of stairs and continue along the narrow path between homes. The atmosphere is tranquil, with the sound of trickling fountains.

- Cross High Tower Dr., which is lined with standalone garages for the residents of the neighborhood's hilltop homes. To the right, you can see the Bolognese-style tower for which the street is named. This structure houses a locked elevator to which only residents have a key. Continue along the path on the other side of High Tower Dr.

- Turn right on Broadview Terrace, another pedestrian path, and continue up the stairs. The homes along this stretch run the gamut from typical Hollywood Mediterranean architecture to modern eclectic. As you approach the tower, notice a raised clearing on your right. This patch of land appears to be too small to accommodate another house and provides a nice vantage point from which to admire the view of Hollywood to the southeast. The hills of Whitley Heights are straight ahead, and the spire of the Capitol Records building pokes up on the other side.

- Ascend the stairs next to High Tower. An interesting, multistory, modern home sits at 2184 Broadview Terrace, next door to the tower.

- Turn right on Alta Loma Terrace, a shady and peaceful path that slopes downward. The houses on either side are accessible only by way of this pathway, hence the detached rows of garages on the street below. Architectural styles range from Mediterranean to Japanese to rambling clapboard farmhouse. This bucolic residential enclave is surrounded by hills, providing isolation from the urban hustle and bustle of the city.

- Turn right to continue along Alta Loma Terrace. You'll come to a charming, fairytale-like house with miniature doors and windows at 6840.

- Turn left to descend the stairs.

- At the bottom of the stairs, you find yourself in a private, fenced-off parking lot for the residents of Alta Loma Terrace. Turn left and head north a short distance to reach the black iron gate exiting onto Highland Ave. on your right.

- On the other side of the gate, turn left on Highland and walk toward the Hollywood Bowl parking lot. Follow the sidewalk adjacent to the lot until you reach the main entrance to the Bowl, which is marked by the 1940 George Stanley Fountain, a beautiful Art Deco piece representing the muse of music.

- Turn left to follow the pathway identified as Peppertree Ln. uphill to the amphitheater. On your left is the Hollywood Bowl Museum. It's worth stopping in to see blown-up panoramic photos of the outdoor theater taken when it was first incorporated into its natural canyon surroundings in 1922, and to admire exhibits about the many legendary performers who have played here over the decades.

- Eventually, you arrive at a circular plaza surrounded by snack bars, the box office, and the Hollywood Bowl gift shop. If there is a concert in session (and you don't have tickets), you won't be able to explore much more. If not, continue up the hill through the turnstiles and enter the massive outdoor venue, which seats nearly 18,000 people. If you're

High Tower

lucky, you might even be able to catch an artist in the middle of sound check. A summer evening at the Bowl is a quintessential LA experience that every resident should try to enjoy at least once a year.

- To leave the Hollywood Bowl complex, return to the plaza in front of the box office and follow the signs for the Odin Lot Path/Museum Terrace, which takes you along an elevated walkway that runs behind the museum and eventually deposits you in the massive parking lot. Just before you descend the stairs to the parking lot, you pass the Museum Terrace patio on your left.

- Turn left to cut through the parking lot back to Highland Ave.

- At Highland, turn right and follow the sidewalk back to Highland-Camrose Park, where you began your walk.

POINTS OF Interest

Hollywood Bowl Museum 2301 N. Highland Ave., Los Angeles, CA 90068, 323-850-2058

route summary

1. Begin at the northwest corner of Highland Ave. and Camrose Dr., and walk northwest through Highland-Camrose Park.

2. Exit the park through the main gateway onto Camrose and turn right

3. Turn right on Rockledge Rd.

4. At the cul-de-sac, you come to Los Altos Pl., a pedestrian walkway. Descend the stairs.

5. Turn right on Broadview Terrace.

6. Ascend the stairs next to High Tower.

7. Turn right on Alta Loma Terrace.

8. Turn right to continue along Alta Loma Terrace.

9. Turn left to descend the stairs.

10. Turn left and head north a short distance to reach the black iron gate exiting onto Highland Ave. on your right.

11. Turn left on Highland Ave. and follow the sidewalk to the main Hollywood Bowl entrance.

12. Turn left at the entrance and follow Peppertree Ln. uphill to the plaza near the box office.

13. If there isn't a concert in session, continue uphill to explore the amphitheater.

14. Return to the plaza in front of the box office and follow the signs for the Odin Lot Path/Museum Terrace.

15. Turn left to cut through the parking lot back to Highland Ave.

16. Turn right to follow the sidewalk back to Highland-Camrose Park.

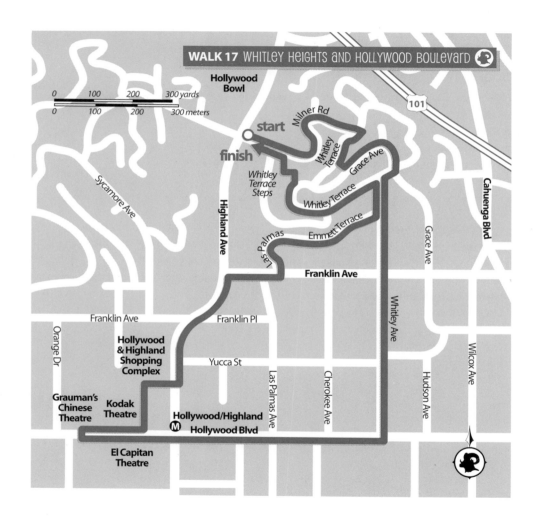

Hollywood Bowl

start

finish

Milner Rd

Whitley Terrace

Grace Ave

Whitley Terrace Steps

Whitley Terrace

Emmett Terrace

Highland Ave

Las Palmas

Franklin Ave

Sycamore Ave

Franklin Ave

Franklin Pl

Yucca St

Grace Ave

Whitley Ave

Cahuenga Blvd

Orange Dr

Hollywood & Highland Shopping Complex

Las Palmas Ave

Cherokee Ave

Hudson Ave

Wilcox Ave

Grauman's Chinese Theatre

Kodak Theatre

Hollywood/Highland
Ⓜ
Hollywood Blvd

El Capitan Theatre

0   100   200   300 yards

0   100   200   300 meters

17 WHITLEY HEIGHTS AND HOLLYWOOD BOULEVARD: A HOLLYWOOD renaissance?

BOUNDARIES: **Hollywood Blvd., Orange Dr., Wilcox Ave., 101 Freeway**
THOMAS GUIDE COORDINATES: **Map 593; E3**
DISTANCE: **Approx. 2 miles**
DIFFICULTY: **Moderate (includes stairways)**
PARKING: **Street parking is available on Milner Rd. (pay attention to posted signs), and there's also a parking lot for the Hollywood Heritage Museum just north of Milner on Highland Ave. Please be aware that parking anywhere in this vicinity on summer evenings can be problematic due to Hollywood Bowl parking restrictions.**
NEAREST METRO STATION: **Hollywood Blvd. and Highland Ave. (Red Line)**

Whitley Heights is a charming, Mediterranean-style residential neighborhood tucked into the hills just east of the Hollywood Bowl. Most of the homes were built between 1918 and 1928, and the predominant architectural style is Spanish Colonial Revival. The seclusion and beauty of this neighborhood attracted such stars as Rudolph Valentino, Judy Garland, and Charlie Chaplin during Hollywood's heyday. Alas, the construction of the 101 Freeway in 1946–47 divided the hill in two, demolishing 40 historic homes in the process. In order to preserve what's left, the Historic Preservation Overlay Zone alliance has granted the neighborhood protected status. Today, Whitley Heights is still home to many industry professionals, and many of the original Mediterranean homes are as lovely as ever, but the address doesn't hold the same prestige it once did.

From Whitley Heights, this route travels down to Hollywood Blvd. and the Hollywood & Highland shopping complex for a glimpse of the newly revitalized heart of Hollywood.

● **Begin on Milner Rd., just east of Highland Ave. and head east, away from Highland. A park that is home to shady picnic areas for Hollywood Bowl patrons, as well as the Hollywood Heritage Museum, is on your left. Pass the Whitley Terrace Steps next door to 6776 Milner (you'll descend these later), and follow the road as it curves to the left, past romantic Mediterranean houses built up against the hill on your right.**

There are charming, cottage-like homes on your left. A posted sign signals that you've entered the Whitley Heights Historical Preservation area.

● Continue uphill and bear right to stay on Milner at the split in the road—you'll notice a stunning white Spanish home on the corner with dark-stained wood and a huge, arched picture window. Two more Spanish Colonial Revival homes catch the eye at 6708 and 6718 Milner; both have a slightly imposing Old World beauty.

● Turn right on Whitley Terrace. Several more elegant, Spanish-style homes adorn the hill on your right. Many of the newer homes in Whitley Heights maintain the Spanish Colonial Revival architectural style, integrating nicely into the old neighborhood. As Whitley Terrace curves to the left, note an interesting, castle-like home at 6697 with unique floral tile murals and stained glass.

● Ascend the hidden wooden staircase on your left, just past 6681 Whitley Terrace. There is a row of standalone garages on the other side of the steps; most of Whitley Heights' homes were built in the 1920s with single-car garages, so the row garages are to accommodate the extra household vehicles.

● Turn left at the top of the steps onto Grace Ave. You're now approaching the upper-most portion of Whitley Heights, where the homes have a peaceful, secluded quality. As you approach the top of the hill, you get a lovely view of Griffith Observatory in the distance. Notice the gated road off to your left, at the point where Grace Ave. turns right. This is Kendra Ct., the only street in the neighborhood that's closed to the public. Continue to follow Grace down the hill.

● When you reach Whitley Terrace, cross the street and continue south down Whitley Ave. This is a tricky four-way intersection, so pay attention to the street signs. Whitley Ave. heads sharply downhill, featuring a mix of old and new apartment buildings. Cross Franklin Ave. and continue south on Whitley as the street levels out. You pass numerous lovely old apartment buildings on this stretch, including the Havenhurst on the southwest corner of Franklin and Whitley; the blue-tiled Hollywood Ardmore, across the street on the southeast corner; the historic Fleur de Lis apartments, at 1825; the self-proclaimed "legendary" Fontenoy Apartments, at 1811; and the La Leyenda building, at 1737. Many of these historic structures feature intricate, wrought-iron fire escape designs and ornately carved stone facades; they recall an elegance that is altogether missing in the mixed-use residential/commercial developments popping up all over Hollywood today.

● Turn right on Hollywood Blvd. and proceed west along the Walk of Fame. While it's true that the boulevard has fallen from its legendary status of the 1920s and '30s, it is currently experiencing a renaissance of sorts. A spattering of notable new attractions combined with the revitalization of many Golden Age landmarks has made Hollywood a viable tourist destination once again.

Hollywood Toys & Costumes, a large shop featuring frightful wigs, sexy costumes, and various props and novelties, is directly ahead, at the end of Whitley Ave. The famous Frederick's of Hollywood Lingerie Museum is right next door; drop in to have a peek at bustiers worn by the likes of Madonna and Cher. Located at 6667 and founded in 1919, Hollywood's oldest restaurant, the Musso & Frank Grill, serves steaks and martinis in a darkened, old-fashioned setting. Built in 1922 as one of Hollywood's original themed movie palaces, the Egyptian Theatre (6712 Hollywood Blvd.) is now owned by the nonprofit film organization American Cinematheque. Next door, the Pig n' Whistle restaurant and bar offers trend-seeking patrons the opportunity to drink and dine on canopied beds.

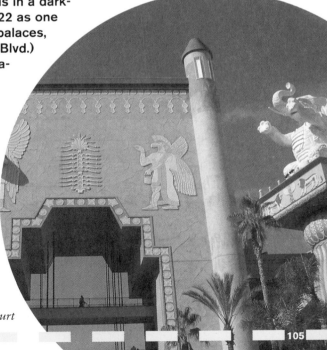

On the north side of the street, at the intersection of McCadden Pl., is the "Artisans Patio," a narrow alley lined with galleries and arts and crafts shops. The Erotic Museum, at 6741 Hollywood Blvd., is open to adults over the age of 18. The lovely, gothic-style First National Bank

Hollywood & Highland's Babylon Court

Building sits on the northeast corner of Hollywood and Highland Ave. Built in 1927, it was designed by Meyer and Holler, the same architectural firm that designed the Grauman's Chinese and Egyptian theaters.

● Cross Highland Ave. The Hollywood & Highland shopping complex occupies a half block on the north side of the street. The brilliantly lit marquee of the El Capitan Theatre (established in 1926) is directly across the street. Today, the former live performance venue shows Disney films, often preceded by a live stage show, making it an exciting destination for kids.

● Take a quick detour west on Hollywood Blvd. to see the Kodak Theatre, which is part of the Hollywood & Highland complex and also the current home of the Academy Awards; the famous Grauman's Chinese Theatre is next door. Built in 1927 and revamped to look a little more contemporary, the lavishly designed (inside and out) theater frequently hosts star-studded movie premieres. The home of the very first Academy Awards ceremony back in 1929, the Hollywood Roosevelt Hotel is just west of the Chinese Theatre on the south side of the street.

● Make your way back to the Hollywood & Highland steps and ascend the wide stairway entrance, which was positioned to provide a framed view of the Hollywood sign in the hills beyond. You'll emerge into Babylon Court, the whimsically named circular plaza at the center of the mall. The bizarre architecture was inspired by D.W. Griffith's 1916 film, *Intolerance*, and features Egyptian imagery from the movie, including giant elephants perched on columns high above Babylon Court. It all makes for an innovative but slightly bewildering shopping environment. Dining options include Vert, Wolfgang Puck's version of a French brasserie; Trastevere, an Italian restaurant; California Pizza Kitchen; and the Grill on Hollywood, a fancy steakhouse. Of course, Hollywood & Highland also features the usual assortment of fashionable clothing and beauty supply and gift stores.

Continue straight through the central plaza and pass under the massive archway, which is decorated with a bas-relief of Egyptian figures. Beyond California Pizza Kitchen, descend the stairs, which will place you in front of the Renaissance Hotel on Highland Ave.

Nearby and Notable

Just northwest of Hollywood & Highland, you'll find two distinctive Hollywood institutions. Built in 1911, the grounds of the Japanese restaurant **Yamashiro** (1999 N. Sycamore Ave., 323-466-5125) were modeled after a palace near Kyoto, and feature acres of lush gardens, as well as a breathtaking view of the city below. **The Magic Castle** (7001 Franklin Ave., 323-851-0800) is located below Yamashiro on the same hill. This exclusive, members-only magic club hosts jaw-dropping performances by talented magicians, but if you want to attend, you have to be invited by a member (a trick that may just require some magic itself).

Located several blocks east of Hollywood & Highland on Hollywood Blvd. is the stunning **Pantages Theatre** (6233 Hollywood Blvd., 323-468-1770). This 1929 Art Deco masterpiece is positively dripping with ornately carved, shimmering, and colorful artistic details—truly a sight to see. The former movie palace now hosts hit Broadway shows and musicals.

● Turn left to head north on Highland, toward the hills. If you look up the hill just to the right of the big church on the northwest corner of Franklin Ave. and Highland, you'll catch a glimpse of one of Frank Lloyd Wright's distinctive Mayan-style textile-block houses.

● Turn right on Franklin Ave. (which comes *after* Franklin Pl.), and pass the corner mall that is home to Whitley Market, which features a small neighborhood grocery store, a flower shop, and, of course, a Starbucks.

● Turn left on Las Palmas Ave. Follow the road as it turns right and becomes Emmet Terrace, a quaint street tucked halfway up the hill. You're now back in Whitley Heights, as evidenced by the abundance of Mediterranean-style hillside homes.

● Turn left on Whitley Ave, ascending the same steep hill you walked down earlier.

● Turn left on Whitley Terrace. A couple of the houses on the left side of the street are modern in design, but most maintain the Mediterranean theme. While the homes on this side of the street appear modestly sized compared with the stately homes on your right, they are actually quite grand, spilling down the hill on the other side and affording spectacular views of Hollywood and beyond.

● Look for the sign for the staircase on your left that reads 2000 N. WHITLEY TERRACE STEPS (just past 6666 Whitley Terrace), and take note of the Hollywood sign in the distance. There is a black wrought-iron gate at the top of the stairs, but it's always unlocked. Descend the long staircase past several homes, a couple of which are only accessible by the stairs, giving them a great feeling of privacy. As you head down, admire the charming vista of the hills on the other side of Highland; the red-tile roofs scattered among the treetops give the impression that you're in a Mediterranean town far from Los Angeles.

You'll encounter another gate at the bottom of the stairway, but, like the gate at the top, it always seems to be unlocked. (In the unlikely case that either gate is locked, you can continue north/northeast on Whitley Terrace, turn left on Milner Rd., and follow the street downhill to your starting point.)

● At the bottom of the steps, turn left on Milner Rd. to return to your starting point.

POINTS OF INTEREST

Hollywood Heritage Museum 2100 N. Highland Ave., Los Angeles, CA 90068, 323-874-4005

Hollywood Toys & Costumes 6600 Hollywood Blvd., Los Angeles, CA 90028, 323-464-4444

Frederick's of Hollywood Lingerie Museum 6608 Hollywood Blvd., Los Angeles, CA 90028, 323-466-8506

Musso & Frank Grill 6667 Hollywood Blvd., Los Angeles, CA 90028, 323-467-7788

Egyptian Theatre 6712 Hollywood Blvd., Los Angeles, CA 90028, 323-466-3456

Pig n' Whistle 6714 Hollywood Blvd., Los Angeles, CA 90028, 323-463-0000

Erotic Museum 6741 Hollywood Blvd., Los Angeles, CA 90028, 323-463-7684

Hollywood & Highland 6801 Hollywood Blvd., Los Angeles, CA 90028, 323-960-2331

El Capitan Theatre 6838 Hollywood Blvd., Los Angeles, CA 90068, 323-467-7674

Kodak Theatre 6801 Hollywood Blvd., Los Angeles, CA 90028, 323-308-6300

Grauman's Chinese Theatre 6925 Hollywood Blvd., Los Angeles, CA 90028, 323-464-6266

route summary

1. Begin on Milner Rd., just east of Highland Ave. and head east.
2. Bear right to stay on Milner at the split in the road.
3. Turn right on Whitley Terrace.
4. Ascend the hidden wooden staircase on your left, just past 6681 Whitley Terrace.
5. Turn left at the top of the steps onto Grace Ave.
6. Cross Whitley Terrace and continue down Whitley Ave.
7. Turn right on Hollywood Blvd.
8. Cross Highland Ave. and continue west for a half block to see Grauman's Chinese Theatre before returning to the stairway leading into the Hollywood & Highland complex just west of Highland Ave.
9. Ascend the stairs into Hollywood & Highland's Babylon Court and continue straight through the mall, descending the stairs back down to Highland Ave.
10. Turn left to head north on Highland.
11. Turn right on Franklin Ave.
12. Turn left on Las Palmas Ave. and follow the road as it turns right and becomes Emmet Terrace.
13. Turn left on Whitley Ave.
14. Turn left on Whitley Terrace.
15. Descend the Whitley Terrace Steps on your left at 2000 N. Whitley.
16. At the bottom of the steps, turn left on Milner Rd. to return to your starting point.

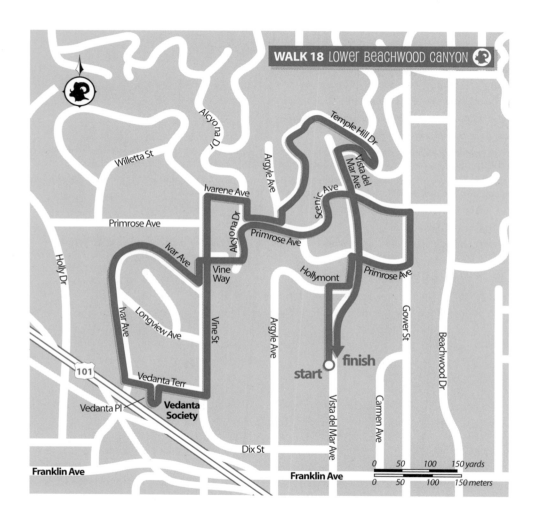

Alcyona Dr

Willetta St

Argyle Ave

Temple Hill Dr

Vista del Mar Ave

Ivarene Ave

Scenic Ave

Primrose Ave

Alcyona Dr

Primrose Ave

Holly Dr

Ivar Ave

Vine Way

Hollymont

Primrose Ave

Vine St

Ivar Ave

Longview Ave

Argyle Ave

Gower St

Beachwood Dr

Vedanta Terr

start

finish

Vista del Mar Ave

Carmen Ave

Vedanta Pl

Vedanta Society

Dix St

Franklin Ave

Franklin Ave

101

| 0 | 50 | 100 | 150 yards |
| 0 | 50 | 100 | 150 meters |

18 LOWER BEACHWOOD CANYON: REMNANTS OF ANCIENT SPIRITUALITY IN THE HOLLYWOOD HILLS

BOUNDARIES: **Franklin Ave., Ivar Ave., Gower St., Temple Hill Dr.**
THOMAS GUIDE COORDINATES: **Map 593; F3**
DISTANCE: **Approx. 2 miles**
DIFFICULTY: **Moderate (includes stairways)**
PARKING: **Free street parking is available on Vista del Mar Ave.**
NEAREST METRO STATION: **Hollywood Blvd. and Vine St. (Red Line)**

You can't get much more "Hollywood" than Beachwood Canyon. Situated in the hills immediately below the legendary sign, this neighborhood is home to rising young stars and accomplished entertainment industry professionals, as well as aging Hollywood burnouts and struggling actors. This disparate community is reflected in the buildings that line the narrow streets, an interesting juxtaposition of beautifully maintained million-dollar-plus houses and rundown '60s-era apartment buildings.

A word of caution to dog walkers: The narrow and winding streets of this hillside neighborhood can be fairly busy; vehicles tend to materialize around blind curves with little advance notice, and sidewalks are scarce. Therefore, it's wise to keep your wits about you and your furry friend on a short leash.

● **Begin on Vista del Mar Ave., north of Franklin Ave., just before the road curves to the right. Straight ahead, you'll see a wide, double staircase.**

● **Ascend the stairway, which was once grand and lovely but has become somewhat dilapidated over the years. At the top of the steps, you see a towering white stucco mansion across the street at 6215 Hollymont Dr. This is the former home of Golden Age actress Barbara Stanwyck. Like the stairway you just ascended, it appears to have fallen from its former glory, but it still stands in reasonably good condition (although one resident has said that it is "very haunted").**

- Turn right on Hollymont and follow it a short distance to Vista del Mar.

- Turn left on Vista del Mar. At 2117–2121 is an apartment building with a sign displaying a pyramid symbol and the words KROTONA OF OLD HOLLYWOOD. This structure is one of several buildings in this area left over from the days of the Krotona Colony, part of the early 20th century Theosophical movement that melded elements of spiritualism, Eastern religion, Masonic lore, and scientific speculation. Across the street is another remnant of the Krotona Colony—the former Krotona Inn, which incorporates elements of Moorish design, particularly in the domed house that is set back from the street amid dense foliage.

- When you reach Primrose Ave., notice the crèche containing a statue of the Madonna and Child on the northeast corner; the cavity has become blackened over the years with the smoke of many candles. Turn right on Primrose and continue for one short block to Gower St.

- Turn left on Gower. At 2122 Gower, look for a small, modern house that incorporates rounded and rectangular shapes to unique effect. The front gate and garage door are painted in primary colors, completing the home's pleasingly kindergarten-like appearance.

NearBY anD NOTaBLe

Franklin Village—located a few blocks east of the starting point of this walk, on Franklin Ave. between Tamarind and Bronson avenues (across the street from the Scientology Celebrity Centre)—is a collection of unique, independently owned businesses that cater to the residents of Beachwood Canyon. The popular strip is home to several decent eateries, such as **Birds**, **Taiyo Sushi**, and **La Poubelle**, as well as the **Bourgeois Pig** coffeehouse, **Real Raw Live** juice bar, **Counterpoint Records & Books**, and the **Upright Citizens Brigade Theater**. (Please refer to the Points of Interest list for business addresses and phone numbers.)

- Upon reaching Scenic Ave., notice the impressive, French Normandy-style apartment complex on the northeast corner. Turn left on Scenic, where the homes are consistently well maintained and attractive, encompassing a variety of architectural styles. A Tudor Revival house, partially obscured by bamboo, sits at 6111 Scenic; directly across the street is an English cottage with an undulating thatched roof.

- Cross Vista del Mar and continue uphill, as the road curves to the left. A flawless Spanish Colonial Revival home in dark-stained wood and pale stucco with intricate tile work catches the eye at 6220.

- Turn right on Primrose Ave., where you'll catch a view to the northwest of a neighborhood known as the Hollywood Knolls in the hills above Lake Hollywood. Cross Argyle Ave. and follow the road downhill.

- Turn left on Alcyona Dr.—a NOT A THROUGH STREET sign makes it easy to spot.

- When you reach the end of the cul-de-sac, keep an eye out for the hidden stairway, and then descend the shady steps to Vine Way.

- Continue straight on Vine Way to Vine St.

- Turn left on Vine St. and follow it one block to Ivar Ave.

- Turn right on Ivar. At 2154 is a wooden, barn-like house that stands out from the other homes in this neighborhood. As Ivar curves around to the left, the street becomes narrow and crowded with parked cars. The sound of rushing traffic indicates that you're approaching the 101 Freeway. At 2062 Ivar, notice the towering home built in the style of a medieval castle.

- Continue past the intersection with Longview Ave., and then turn left on Vedanta Terrace, immediately before the freeway overpass.

- When you reach the intersection with Vedanta Pl., turn right to take a quick detour to the Vedanta Society of Southern California complex, which features a bookstore and a white temple that looks like a mini Taj Mahal. The Vedanta Society is an ancient religious philosophy based on the sacred scriptures of India known as the Vedas.

The temple is open to the public daily for meditation, classes, lectures, and seminars. After checking out the temple, return to Vedanta Terrace and turn right.

- Turn left on Vine St. and look over your shoulder to the south to see the top of the distinctive Capitol Records building on the other side of the freeway. At 2030 Vine is a lovely Spanish Mission-style home with a little bell set into the arch over the front gate. A fountain can be heard trickling inside the hidden courtyard. Another charming Spanish-style residence, the Monastery Gardens apartments, is situated a little farther up the street, at 2062.

- Turn right on Ivarene Ave. A brilliant, golden-colored stucco home sits at 6281 Ivarene.

- To the left of the intersection of Alcyona Dr., at 2174 Alcyona, notice the remarkable house constructed of weathered wooden boards—it looks like a mountain ski lodge incongruously set in the heavily Mediterranean-influenced Hollywood Hills. Turn right on Alcyona.

- Turn left on Primrose Ave., heading back up the steep hill you descended earlier.

- Turn left on Argyle Ave. at the top of the hill.

- Turn right on Temple Hill Dr. On the northeast corner, notice the blue-shingled farmhouse that is almost completely obscured by bushes and trees. Temple Hill Dr. has a rustic air—it's so high in the hills that the freeway and the sordid streets of Hollywood seem far away.

- As the road curves downhill, there are fewer houses, emphasizing the rural feel, until an unexpected view of downtown Los Angeles materializes as the road turns to the southeast.

- Turn right on Vista del Mar Ave., where Temple Hill ends. Continue downhill along the curving street, and take note of the various architectural styles—Spanish, English, Tudor, Moorish, modern; the residents of the Hills have no compunction about mixing and matching their architectural styles, but the effect is more whimsical than tacky. At the intersection with Vista del Mar Pl., turn left to stay on Vista del Mar Ave. Cross

Scenic Ave. and Primrose Ave., retracing your steps down to Hollymont. Instead of turning on Hollymont to descend the stairway from the beginning of the walk, remain on Vista del Mar as it curves to the right, taking you back to the beginning of your journey.

If you're feeling peckish, you can continue one block south to the 101 Coffee Shop, a casual, vaguely retro-themed neighborhood eatery inside the motel on the corner of Vista del Mar and Franklin Ave.

POINTS OF INTEREST

Vedanta Society of Southern California 1946 Vedanta Pl., Hollywood, CA 90068, 323-465-7114

101 Coffee Shop 6145 Franklin Ave., Los Angeles, CA 90028, 323-467-1175

Bourgeois Pig 5931 Franklin Ave., Los Angeles, CA 90028, 323-464-6008

Birds 5925 Franklin Ave., Los Angeles, CA 90028, 323-465-0175

Upright Citizens Brigade Theater 5919 Franklin Ave., Los Angeles, CA 90028, 323-908-8702

Taiyo Sushi 5917 Franklin Ave., Los Angeles, CA 90028, 323-468-2496

Real Raw Live 5913 Franklin Ave. Los Angeles, CA 90028, 323-461-4545

Counterpoint Records & Books 5911 Franklin Ave., Los Angeles, CA 90028, 323-957-7965

La Poubelle 5907 Franklin Ave., Los Angeles, CA 90028, 323-465-0807

route summary

1. Head north on Vista del Mar Ave. and ascend the staircase (don't follow the road as it curves to the right).
2. Turn right on Hollymont Dr.
3. Turn left on Vista del Mar Ave.
4. Turn right on Primrose Ave.
5. Turn left on Gower St.
6. Turn left on Scenic Ave.
7. Turn right on Primrose Ave.
8. Turn left on Alcyona Dr.
9. Descend the stairway to Vine Way.
10. Continue straight on Vine Way.
11. Turn left on Vine St.
12. Turn right on Ivar Ave.
13. Turn left on Vedanta Terrace.
14. Turn right on Vedanta Pl.
15. Return to Vedanta Terrace and turn right.
16. Turn left on Vine St.
17. Turn right on Ivarene Ave.
18. Turn right on Alcyona Dr.
19. Turn left on Primrose Ave.
20. Turn left on Argyle Ave.
21. Turn right on Temple Hill Dr.
22. Turn right on Vista del Mar Ave.
23. Turn left to stay on Vista del Mar Ave. (avoiding Vista del Mar Pl.).
24. Follow Vista del Mar Ave. as it curves to the right, taking you downhill to the beginning of your walk

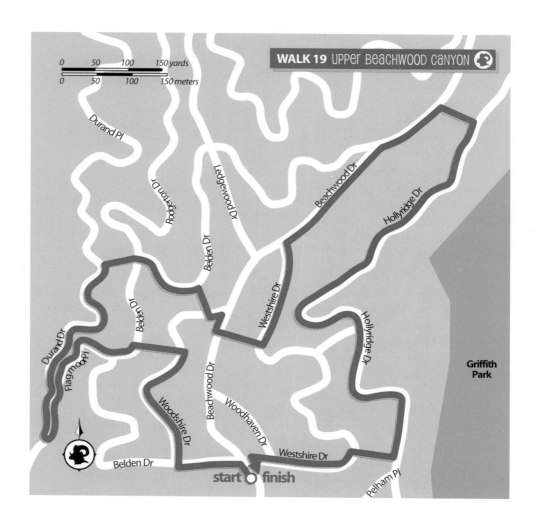

0   50   100   150 yards
0   50   100   150 meters

Durand Pl

Rodgerton Dr

Ledgewood Dr

Belden Dr

Beachwood Dr

Hollyridge Dr

Westshire Dr

Hollyridge Dr

Griffith Park

Durand Dr

Flagmoor Pl

Belden Dr

Woodshire Dr

Beachwood Dr

Woodhaven Dr

Westshire Dr

Belden Dr

start • finish

Pelham Pl

19 Upper Beachwood Canyon: Home Sweet Hollywood Home

BOUNDARIES: **Franklin Ave., 101 Freeway, Griffith Park**
THOMAS GUIDE COORDINATES: **Map 593; F1/G1**
DISTANCE: **Approx. 2 miles**
DIFFICULTY: **Strenuous (includes stairways)**
PARKING: **Free parking is available on Beachwood Dr.**

Beachwood Canyon works hard to maintain its rural, small-town vibe, even though its population is about as Hollywood as you can get. The neighborhood's origins reflect this conceit; in 1923, real estate magnate S.H. Woodruff developed the rustic hills north of Hollywood, which he topped off with an ostentatious, four-story sign dubbing it "Hollywoodland." The last four letters have since been removed, and the remainder of the sign—now one of the most recognizable Southern California landmarks in the world—has been treated to the occasional facelift over the past 80 years (this is Hollywood, after all).

At the time of development, Woodruff hired European stonemasons to construct roadside walls and six long stairways out of wrought iron and stone to interconnect the residential streets of Hollywoodland. This walk seeks out and conquers every one of these steep flights, so be sure to bring plenty of water and wear comfy shoes.

● Begin on Beachwood Dr., just south of Belden Dr. (which is called Westshire Dr. to the east of Beachwood), and head north into the canyon. The original stone gates of Hollywoodland sit on either side of the road, and a street sign welcomes residents home while imploring them to "slow down and relax." To the right, at 2700 Westshire Dr., is the original Hansel-and-Gretel-style cottage that still houses the Hollywoodland Realty Company.

● Turn left on Belden Dr. and walk past the neighborhood hub, where locals grab breakfast at the Village Coffee Shop, do light grocery shopping at the Beachwood Market, and stay current on the community happenings posted on the neighborhood bulletin board.

- Turn right on Woodshire Dr., a narrow, winding street with a pleasing rustic feel, which you follow past flawless Spanish homes, many with stained-glass details in the windows. An imposing Norman castle-style home at 2755 Woodshire catches the eye. Next door is an ivy-covered English cottage with a coat of arms painted over the front door. While the predominant architectural style in the canyon is Mediterranean, the Anglo influence is also apparent.

- Just before 2795 Woodshire, look for the first of the somewhat hidden Hollywoodland stairways on your left and ascend it.

- Emerge back on Belden Dr. and turn left.

- When you reach the fork in the road, bear right to continue uphill on Flagmoor Pl. About halfway up the short street, a clearing on the left treats you to a great view of downtown's high-rises to the southeast. And as you approach the next intersection, you can catch an unobstructed view of Griffith Observatory directly to the east.

- At the intersection of Flagmoor Pl. and Durand Dr., bear left slightly to head uphill on Durand. You'll notice a great stone wall on your right. Follow this to the front of the magnificent home at 2869 Durand, which was built in the style of a French chateau.

- Cross in front of the entrance to 2869 Durand, and take a few steps down the dirt trail that lies next to the small, private parking area. The Lake Hollywood Reservoir sparkles below.

- Retrace your steps from the trail back to Durand Dr., and turn left on Durand—back the way you came. Now heading north, you pass the intersection with Flagmoor Pl. The Hollywood sign looms large directly ahead.

- Just past 2954 Durand is the second stairway, which is broken up by pathways and landings. Follow the steps all the way down to the street below. Use caution, as some of the stairs have eroded over time. As you descend, you'll see a large, rectilinear modern home dead ahead; this is another common architectural style in these hills. At the bottom of the steps, cross Rodgerton Dr. to continue straight on Belden Dr.

- Follow Belden as it curves around, and look for the next stairway, just past 2950 Belden. This straight, narrow flight, divided by what used to be small ponds but are now sand-filled planters, is perhaps the most recognizable stairway in Beachwood Canyon. Descend the steps, and then turn left on Woodshire Dr. at the bottom. A bronze Los Angeles Cultural Heritage Commission sign at the base declares Hollywoodland's granite retaining walls and interconnecting stairways as historic cultural monuments.

- Cross Beachwood Dr. and turn right on the other side of the street. Between 2800 and 2810 Beachwood is another very long stairway. Take a deep breath and ascend the 144 steps to Westshire Dr. Again, watch out for cracks and holes in the 80-year-old concrete.

- Turn left at the top of the stairs and follow Westshire Dr. downhill to where it merges with Beachwood Dr.

- Continue north on Beachwood, past vibrantly painted Spanish homes, charming traditional wood-and-brick houses, and faux castles—the residence at 2925 even features a large mural of a medieval knight on the wall facing the street. As you approach the intersection with Belden Dr., notice the particularly adorable English cottage at 2958, complete with low stone walls and a thatched-style roof.

- Cross Belden Dr. and continue on Beachwood, keeping an eye out for the next staircase, which lies between 3020 and 3030 Beachwood. Begin your ascent up the longest stairway of this walk—176 steps—pausing as needed to catch

Hollywoodland gates

your breath. The houses on either side have particularly large lots, lending a nice, open feel to this portion of the walk.

- At the top of the stairs, turn right on Hollyridge Dr. for the longest stairway-free stretch of this route. Thankfully, the road slopes gently downhill here, providing some relief after the grueling sets of stairs you have climbed. Many of the homes on the hill to your left are concealed behind dense foliage, but you can catch glimpses of several interesting styles, including another stone castle and a few starkly modern residences. There's a fine line between eccentric and tacky, and you may agree that some of the architecture in the canyon walks that line. Continue straight on Hollyridge past the intersection with Lechner Pl.

- At the intersection with Pelham Pl., just past 2831 Hollyridge, turn right to descend the final stairway of your journey.

- At the bottom of the steps, turn left to follow Westshire Dr. for about a block back to Beachwood Dr., and then turn left to return to your starting point next to the stone gates marking the entrance to Hollywoodland.

POINTS OF INTEREST

Village Coffee Shop 2695 N. Beachwood Dr., Los Angeles, CA 90068, 323-467-5398
Beachwood Market 2701 Belden Dr., Los Angeles, CA 90068, 323-464-7154

route summary

1.   Begin on Beachwood Dr., just south of Belden Dr. and head north.

2.   Turn left on Belden Dr.

3.   Turn right on Woodshire Dr.

4.   Ascend the stairway just before 2795 Woodshire.

5.   At the top, turn left on Belden Dr.

6.   Bear right to continue uphill on Flagmoor Pl.

7.   At the intersection with Durand Dr., bear left slightly to continue uphill on Durand.

8.   Cross in front of the entrance to 2869 Durand, and take a few steps down the dirt trail that lies next to the parking area for a view of the Lake Hollywood Reservoir below.

9.   Retrace your steps from the trail back to Durand Dr., and turn left—back the way you came—to head north on Durand, passing the intersection with Flagmoor Pl.

10.   Just past 2954 Durand, descend the next set of stairs.

11.   At the bottom of the steps, cross Rodgerton Dr. to continue straight on Belden Dr.

12.   Descend the stairway just past 2950 Belden and turn left on Woodshire Dr. at the bottom.

13.   Cross Beachwood Dr. and turn right on the other side of the street to ascend the stairway between 2800 and 2810 Beachwood Dr.

14.   At the top of the stairs, turn on Westshire Dr. and follow it downhill to where the road merges with Beachwood Dr.

15.   Continue north on Beachwood.

16.   Ascend the staircase between 3020 and 3030 Beachwood Dr.

17.   At the top of the stairs, turn right on Hollyridge Dr.

18.   At the intersection with Pelham Pl., just past 2831 Hollyridge, turn right to descend the stairs.

19.   At the bottom of the steps, turn left to follow Westshire Dr. for about a block back to Beachwood Dr.

20.   Turn left on Beachwood to return to your starting point.

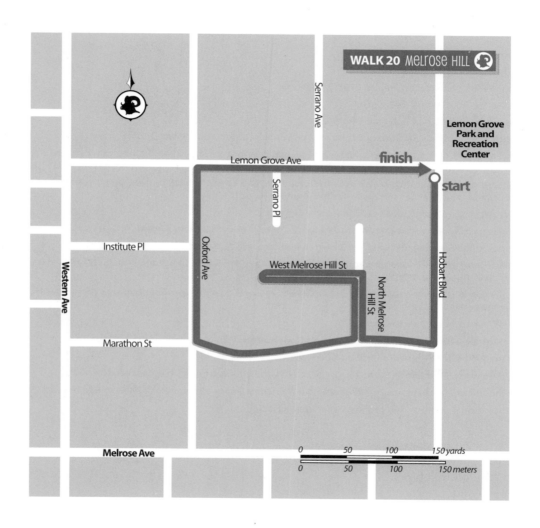

WALK 20 MELROSE HILL

Lemon Grove Park and Recreation Center

Serrano Ave

Lemon Grove Ave

finish

start

Serrano Pl

Institute Pl

Oxford Ave

West Melrose Hill St

North Melrose Hill St

Hobart Blvd

Western Ave

Marathon St

Melrose Ave

| 0 | 50 | 100 | 150 yards |
| 0 | 50 | 100 | 150 meters |

20 MeLrOSe HILL: DIaMOND IN THe rOUGH

BOUNDARIES: Western Ave., Melrose Ave., Lemon Grove Ave., Hobart Blvd.
THOMAS GUIDE COORDINATES: Map 593: H6
DISTANCE: Approx. ½ mile
DIFFICULTY: Easy
PARKING: Free street parking is available on Lemon Grove Ave. and Hobart Blvd.

Melrose Hill is an easy place to miss, which is a shame. This small but notable neighborhood is situated in the heavily urban area just north of Melrose Ave. and east of Western Ave. This region's proximity to these busy thoroughfares, not to mention the adjacent 101 Freeway, contributes to the somewhat grimy atmosphere.

But the two cross streets that comprise Melrose Hill seem far removed from their surroundings and are worth exploring. Los Angeles' Historic Preservation Overlay Zone alliance also thinks so, and the organization granted this neighborhood historic status for the architectural significance of its California bungalows, which incorporate elements of both Craftsman and Colonial Revival styles. No more than a half mile from start to finish, this trek essentially amounts to a walk around the block and focuses on the charming and distinctive homes atop the hill.

- Begin at the corner of Lemon Grove Ave. and Hobart Blvd. The Lemon Grove Park and Recreation Center sits on the northeast corner of this intersection, and you can catch a lovely view of the Griffith Observatory to the north.

- Head south on Hobart Blvd. This street is home to mostly Latino families, and you're likely to see kids playing in the front yards as their parents look on.

- Turn right on Marathon St. In contrast to Hobart, which sees its share of traffic, this street is peaceful, becoming quieter still as it slopes gently uphill. The tidily kept bungalows on this block have a timeless beauty; they seem out of place in the middle of Hollywood.

- Turn right on N. Melrose Hill St. As is typical in Los Angeles, the houses are slightly larger as you move farther uphill.

- Turn left on W. Melrose Hill St. On the southwest corner of 4900 W. Melrose Hill and 800 N. Melrose Hill is a gorgeous, dark wood, shingle-and-brick house.

- Continue to the end of the cul-de-sac, taking a minute to admire the classic Craftsman home at 4954 and the unique American Colonial Revival house next door, at 4960.

- Make your way back to the intersection of N. Melrose Hill, and turn right to retrace your steps to Marathon.

- Turn right on Marathon. Part of what makes this neighborhood so delightful is its abundance of trees; the sidewalk is shaded with palms, jacaranda trees, and crepe myrtle.

- Turn right on Oxford Ave. The large, wood-sided houses on your right appear to be older, or perhaps just not as well maintained, as the homes on Melrose Hill.

- Turn right on Lemon Grove Ave. You may want to take a short detour to peruse the attractive, Spanish-style apartments at the end of the short cul-de-sac at Serrano Pl. Many of the homes on Lemon Grove have bars on the windows, a reminder that this isn't the safest neighborhood in LA. But it's by far not the most dangerous, either.

- Return to your starting point at the intersection of Lemon Grove and Hobart Blvd.

route summary

1. Begin at the corner of Lemon Grove Ave. and Hobart Blvd. and head south on Hobart.
3. Turn right on Marathon St.
4. Turn right on N. Melrose Hill St.
5. Turn left on W. Melrose Hill St.
6. Continue to the end of the cul-de-sac, and then retrace your steps back to N. Melrose Hill.
7. Turn right on N. Melrose Hill to retrace your steps back to Marathon St.
8. Turn right on Marathon St.
9. Turn right on Oxford Ave.
10. Turn right on Lemon Grove Ave.
11. Return to the start at the intersection of Lemon Grove Ave. and Hobart Blvd.

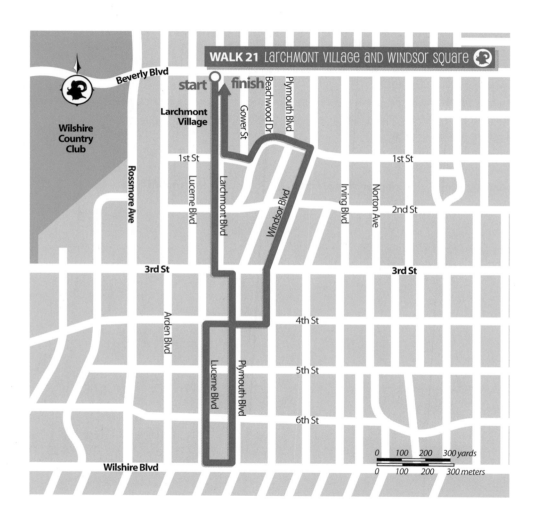

WALK 21 LarCHMONT VILLage anD WinDSor SQuare

Beverly Blvd

start finish

Larchmont Village

Wilshire Country Club

Rossmore Ave

Gower St

Beechwood Dr

Plymouth Blvd

1st St

1st St

Lucerne Blvd

Larchmont Blvd

Windsor Blvd

Irving Blvd

Norton Ave

2nd St

3rd St

3rd St

Arden Blvd

4th St

Lucerne Blvd

Plymouth Blvd

5th St

6th St

Wilshire Blvd

0   100   200   300 yards
0   100   200   300 meters

128

21 Larchmont Village and Windsor Square: a welcome dose of small-town charm

BOUNDARIES: **Beverly Blvd., Rossmore Ave., Wilshire Blvd., Windsor Blvd.**
THOMAS GUIDE COORDINATES: **Map 633; F1**
DISTANCE: **Approx. 2 miles**
DIFFICULTY: **Easy**
PARKING: **Free street parking is available on Larchmont Blvd., south of 1st St.; there is metered parking on Larchmont north of 1st St.**

The Hancock Park/Windsor Square region lies just south of Hollywood and is considered one of the nicest areas in central Los Angeles. It encompasses posh Wilshire Country Club, as well as Larchmont Village, a collection of small, independently owned shops and restaurants (as well as a few commercial chain establishments) that is constantly teeming with residents and their canine companions. This route begins in the Village and heads south to explore the ostentatious homes of Windsor Square, a wealthy neighborhood that the city of Los Angeles declared a Historic Preservation Overlay Zone (HPOZ) in 2005. There was some dispute among the residents of Windsor Square over this declaration. The HPOZ designation can be a blessing in that it protects the houses and ensures that the architectural integrity and cohesiveness of all the buildings in that area are carefully upheld, but it can also be limiting to residents who wish to impose their own unique mark on their property.

● Begin at the corner of Beverly Blvd. and Larchmont Blvd., in the middle of Larchmont Village, which stretches for several blocks between Melrose Ave. and 3rd St. Head south on Larchmont. The Village is home to more restaurants than you can shake a fork at, ranging from Italian to Greek to Thai to Caribbean. It also features such commercial staples as Starbucks, Baskin-Robbins, and Jamba Juice. Sartorial enthusiasts will be delighted to find a collection of fine boutiques along Larchmont, although the names on some of the storefronts seem to change regularly. It's worth your time either before or after this walk to explore Larchmont Village and grab a bite to eat—if you can make up your mind about where to dine. Dependable eateries include Chan Dara (a popular Thai restaurant just north of Beverly Blvd.), Prado Restaurant, Cafe du Village, Village Pizzeria, and Le Petit Greek.

Larchmont Blvd. becomes a residential street south of 1st St., populated with mostly Spanish and Norman one- and two-story homes. The street median is planted with flowering trees, lily of the Nile, and bird of paradise. On the southwest corner of 2nd St. and Larchmont, notice a wood-shingled home with an eye-catching, Polynesian-themed garden dominated by a lacquered red bridge and wishing well. The Japanese-inspired wishing well, decorated with a picture of Snow White and the words, "I'm wishing," would be incongruous anywhere but LA. As it turns out, this house was designed and built by Adriana Caselotti, who provided the voice of Snow White in the 1937 animated feature. After lending her voice to the raven-haired cartoon character (a tribute to her human counterpart, as Snow White was originally conceived to have blond hair), Caselotti taught singing lessons in Hawaii and came to love Asian culture, hence the idiosyncratically designed home and garden.

As you near 3rd St., look for the stone column erected by the Windsor Square Association at the south end of the Larchmont median.

● Cross 3rd St. and then turn left, walking less than a block to Plymouth Blvd.

● Turn right on Plymouth, a quiet street lined with royal palms. The houses here are more appropriately described as mansions, with expansive green lawns and self-conscious ornamentation such as diamond-paned windows and gingerbread trim. The primary architectural styles are those that work well on a grand scale, such as American Colonial Revival, Spanish Colonial Revival, and Tudor Revival. The house at 425 Plymouth is notable for its pale green tile roof—a rare deviation from the typical red clay tiles—and Corinthian-style columns upholding the front entryway. After crossing 6th St., you'll pass the Windsor House at 606 Plymouth Blvd.; the imposing brick Tudor building is securely gated off from the street and is the official residence of the Los Angeles mayor.

● Turn right on Wilshire Blvd. The commanding structure of the Scottish Rite Masonic Temple sits on the northwest corner of Plymouth and Wilshire. The temple houses the American Heritage Masonic Museum, which celebrates the humanitarian and academic influence of Freemasons throughout history. On the south side of Wilshire is the Wilshire United Methodist Church, a beautiful building that combines elements of Romanesque and Gothic design and has been declared a historic cultural monument by the city of Los Angeles. The Italian Renaissance-style headquarters for the Ebell of Los Angeles, just west of the church, at the corner of Lucerne Blvd., encompasses the Wilshire Ebell Theatre and Clubhouse. Founded in 1894, the Ebell of Los Angeles is one of the nation's oldest and largest women's clubs. The theater and clubhouse were built in 1927.

- Turn right on Lucerne Blvd. At 637 Lucerne, take note of a Victorian mansion. Across the street, at 630, is an elaborate Craftsman shingled in dark green wood. Apart from these two remarkable structures, most of the homes along Lucerne echo the same architectural styles on Plymouth.

- Turn right on 4th St., and note the lovely white mansion on the southeast corner of Lucerne and 4th.

- Turn left on Windsor Blvd. A classic white American Colonial Revival home sits on the northeast corner at 354 Windsor.

- Carefully cross 3rd St.; the street is fairly busy and there's no crosswalk at Windsor. At 270 S. Windsor, a cheerful orange Spanish home with blue-and-white-striped awnings catches the eye. As you continue along Windsor, you'll see that many of the gardens are planted with white roses and purple lily of the Nile; the landscaping along this street is impressively congruous. As you cross 2nd St., notice the magnificent live oak tree stretching its low, dense branches across the sidewalk on the northeast corner. Even in the dry heat of summer, Windsor Blvd. smells verdant, thanks to the blooming magnolia trees and amply watered lawns.

- Turn left on 1st St. The Spanish-style home on the northwest corner looks like a tropical resort, gorgeously landscaped with palms and exotic flowering plants. As you cross Plymouth Blvd. for the last time, look to the north to catch a glimpse of the water tower at Paramount Studios.

- When you come to the intersection of Beachwood Dr., veer left to remain on 1st St., crossing Gower St. and returning to the intersection of Larchmont Blvd.

- Turn right on Larchmont and head one block back to Beverly Blvd., where you started in Larchmont Village.

POINTS OF INTErEST

Chan Dara Restaurant 310 N. Larchmont Blvd., Los Angeles, CA 90004, 323-467-1052

Prado Restaurant 244 N. Larchmont Blvd., Los Angeles, CA 90004, 323-467-3871

Cafe du Village 139½ N. Larchmont Blvd., Los Angeles, CA 90004, 323-466-3996

Village Pizzeria 131 N. Larchmont Blvd., Los Angeles, CA 90004, 323-465-5566

Le Petit Greek 127 N. Larchmont Blvd., Los Angeles, CA 90004, 323-464-5160

American Heritage Masonic Museum 4357 Wilshire Blvd., Los Angeles, CA 90010, 323-930-9806

Ebell Club of Los Angeles 743 S. Lucerne Blvd., Los Angeles, CA 90005, 323-931-1277

route summary

1. Begin at the corner of Beverly Blvd. and Larchmont Blvd. and head south on Larchmont.
2. Cross 3rd St. and then turn left.
3. Turn right on Plymouth Blvd.
4. Turn right on Wilshire Blvd.
5. Turn right on Lucerne Blvd.
6. Turn right on 4th St.
7. Turn left on Windsor Blvd.
8. Turn left on 1st St.
9. At the intersection of Beachwood Dr., veer left to remain on 1st St.
10. Turn right on Larchmont Blvd. and head one block to Beverly Blvd., where this walk began.

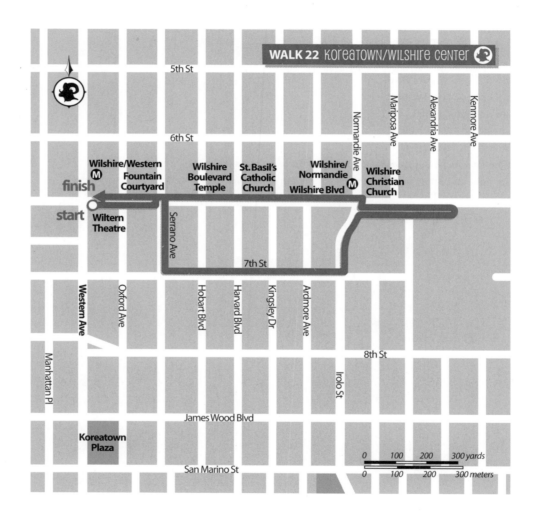

5th St

6th St

Mariposa Ave

Alexandria Ave

Kenmore Ave

Normandie Ave

Wilshire/Western
Fountain
Courtyard

Wilshire
Boulevard
Temple

St. Basil's
Catholic
Church

Wilshire/
Normandie

Wilshire Christian
Church

finish

start

Wiltern
Theatre

Wilshire Blvd

Serrano Ave

7th St

Western Ave

Oxford Ave

Hobart Blvd

Harvard Blvd

Kingsley Dr

Ardmore Ave

8th St

Irolo St

Manhattan Pl

James Wood Blvd

Koreatown
Plaza

San Marino St

0   100   200   300 yards
0   100   200   300 meters

22 Koreatown/Wilshire Center: Contemporary Korean Culture Meets Los Angeles History

BOUNDARIES: **Western Ave., Wilshire Blvd., Catalina St., 7th St.**
THOMAS GUIDE COORDINATES: **Map 633; H2**
DISTANCE: **Approx. 1½ miles**
DIFFICULTY: **Easy**
PARKING: **Metered street parking is available on Western Ave.**
NEAREST METRO STATION: **Wilshire Blvd. and Western Ave., or Wilshire Blvd. and Normandie Ave. (Purple Line)**

The area known as Koreatown or Wilshire Center truly has it all—historical buildings, a plethora of dining and shopping options, a giant spa and sports club, and a sizzling night scene. The neighborhood even features two convenient Metro stations, making it easy to get here and spend both day and night without worrying about parking fees (or designating a driver, should that become an issue). While the area is home to a mostly Korean-American population and many of the businesses cater primarily to Korean-speaking clientele, it has plenty to offer anyone else looking for an adventure, a dose of Los Angeles history, or a taste of authentic Korean culture.

● Begin at the corner of Wilshire Blvd. and Western Ave. The Wilshire/Western Metro station is located at the northeast corner, and the striking Wiltern Theatre building is directly across the street. This green terra-cotta Art Deco structure opened as an office building and movie theater in 1931, and has since been renovated and declared a Los Angeles Historic Cultural Monument. Today the venue hosts a variety of performances, from comedy acts to garage bands. Take a minute to check out the underside of the flashy metal and neon marquee, which is decorated with an ornate sunburst design in plaster, and the beautiful carved mahogany doors of the theater lobby.

Head east on the south side of Wilshire, passing Opus Bar & Grill, a posh nightspot occupying the former space of the retro-style jazz supper club Atlas. Opus serves "modern California" steak and seafood and boasts one of the largest bars in Los Angeles.

The Aroma Spa and Sports Center occupies the southeast corner of the intersection with Serrano Ave.; its *Blade Runner*-esque electronic billboard lures passersby to try out the exclusive club's saunas, spa treatments, four-story driving range, and other sports facilities.

● Cross to the north side of Wilshire Blvd. at Serrano and continue east. You'll pass the Wilshire Boulevard Temple on the northeast corner of Wilshire and Hobart. Built in 1929, this striking Byzantine-influenced structure is listed in the U.S. Register of Historic Places. The building's exterior is dominated by a massive dome 100 feet in diameter. If the synagogue is open to the public at the time of your visit, take time to explore inside, which is decorated in gold and black Italian marble and features murals depicting the biblical story of creation.

After crossing Harvard Blvd. you'll come upon St. Basil's Catholic Church (established in 1969), an imposing building whose vertical concrete panels are interspersed with jagged columns of colorful stained glass, giving it the slightly discordant feel of a Picasso painting.

BCD Tofu House is located on the southeast corner of Wilshire and Kingsley Dr. Here you can get a table full of *banchan* (assorted Korean salads and pickles) to go with your delicious bubbling bowl of *soon* (a flavorful stew served with tofu and your choice of meat, fish, or vegetables), all for under $10. It's even open 24 hours.

● At the northeast corner of Wilshire and Normandie Ave. is the Wilshire Christian Church, an ornate Romanesque structure built in 1927. Cross Normandie and then cross to the south side of Wilshire, and continue east. From this side of the street, you have a better view of the white Art Deco building just east of Wilshire Christian Church, which houses the Consulate General of the Republic of Indonesia. On your right, pass a variety of small, inexpensive eateries. This area is bustling with office workers on the weekdays; worthwhile lunch spots here include Wasabi for Japanese food, Mamma Mia for Italian, and Cafe Metro for toasted sandwiches and hearty salads.

After crossing Mariposa Ave., note Wilshire Center's tallest structure, the Equitable Life Building, which towers over the opposite side of the boulevard. The Wilshire Center Farmers Market takes place on Mariposa north of Wilshire every Friday from 11:30 A.M. to 3 P.M., and is a wonderful place to pick up lunch, produce, nuts, flowers, and miscellaneous items like handbags and designer jeans of questionable authenticity.

The northeast corner of Wilshire and Alexandria Ave. is the former site of the first of the legendary hat-shaped Brown Derby restaurants, but the site is now occupied by a cheesy-looking strip mall (named "Brown Derby Plaza" in honor of the former Hollywood Golden Age hot spot). Just east of the plaza are the 1920s-era Gaylord Apartments, named for Henry Gaylord Wilshire, the millionaire who developed what is now called MacArthur Park (located in a former high-crime but slowly gentrifying neighborhood a little over a mile east of here). According to popular lore, Wilshire Blvd. was so-named because Wilshire would only allow a boulevard to bisect his property if it bore his name.

On the south side of the street is the former site of the Ambassador Hotel, the legendary playground for Hollywood's rich and famous and the infamous site of Robert F. Kennedy's assassination. The hotel and its Cocoanut Grove nightclub opened in 1921 and enjoyed decades of fame as a beautiful people's mecca before Sirhan Sirhan killed Robert F. Kennedy at the

Wilshire Blvd.

Ambassador on June 5, 1968. The hotel was demolished in 2006, and the property now belongs to the Los Angeles Unified School District. A sign on the street median declares this stretch of Wilshire Blvd. to be the Robert F. Kennedy Memorial Parkway.

- Retrace your steps to Normandie Ave., and turn left on Normandie/Irolo St. Another historic apartment building, the Piccadilly, is located at 682 S. Irolo St.

- Turn right on 7th St., a residential street occupied, for the most part, by anonymous apartment buildings. One notable exception is the cute apartment building at 3530 W. 7th St.—its rounded corners and retro, '50s-style architecture bring to mind the fenders of a classic automobile.

- Turn right on Serrano Ave. You'll notice the netted driving range of Aroma Spa and Sports on your right. The Koreatown branch of the Los Angeles public library is on your left.

- Cross Wilshire Blvd. and turn left. The curved twin towers of the Wilshire Colonnade office complex on your right are built around a gorgeous circular fountain courtyard—a nice place to enjoy a sandwich or an iced coffee from the Starbucks across the street.

- Continue for two blocks to your starting point at the corner of Wilshire and Western.

POINTS OF INTEREST

Wiltern Theatre 3790 Wilshire Blvd., Los Angeles, CA 90010, 213-380-5005

Opus Bar & Grill 3760 Wilshire Blvd., Los Angeles, CA 90010, 213-738-1600

Aroma Spa and Sports 3680 Wilshire Blvd., Los Angeles, CA 90010, 213-387-0212

Wilshire Boulevard Temple 3663 Wilshire Blvd., Los Angeles, CA 90010, 213-388-2401

St. Basil's Catholic Church 3611 Wilshire Blvd., Los Angeles, CA 90010, 213-381-6191

BCD Tofu House 3575 Wilshire Blvd., Los Angeles, CA 90010, 213-382-6677

Wilshire Christian Church 634 S. Normandie Ave., Los Angeles, CA 90005, 213-382-6337

Wilshire Center Farmers Market Mariposa Ave. just north of Wilshire Blvd., Los Angeles, CA 90005, Fridays 11:30 A.M. to 3 P.M.

route summary

1. Begin at the corner of Wilshire Blvd. and Western Ave. and head east on the south side of Wilshire.

2. Cross to the north side of Wilshire Blvd. at Serrano Ave. and continue to head east.

3. Cross to the east side of Normandie and then cross back to the south side of Wilshire and continue to head east to Alexandria Ave.

4. Retrace your steps to Normandie Ave. and turn left on Normandie/Irolo St.

5. Turn right on 7th St.

6. Turn right on Serrano Ave.

7. Cross Wilshire Blvd. and turn left.

8. Continue for two blocks to your starting point at the corner of Wilshire and Western.

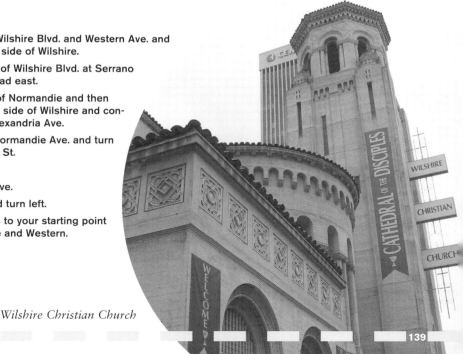

Wilshire Christian Church

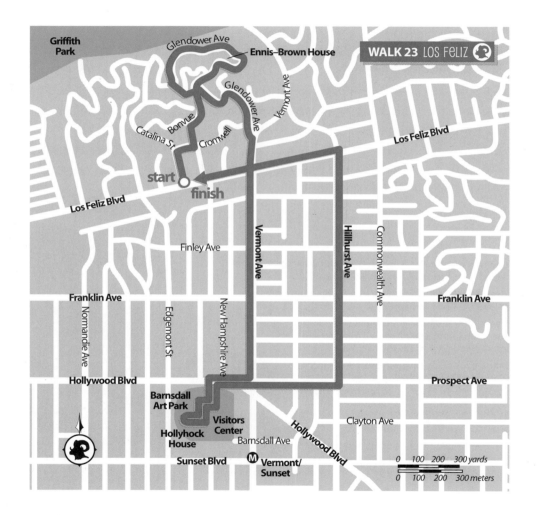

Griffith
Park

Glendower Ave

Ennis–Brown House

Vermont Ave

Glendower Ave

Catalina St

Bonvue

Cromwell

WALK 23 LOS FELIZ

Los Feliz Blvd

start

finish

Los Feliz Blvd

Finley Ave

Vermont Ave

Hillhurst Ave

Commonwealth Ave

Franklin Ave

Franklin Ave

Normandie Ave

Edgemont St

New Hampshire Ave

Hollywood Blvd

**Barnsdall
Art Park**

Prospect Ave

Clayton Ave

**Visitors
Center**

**Hollyhock
House**

Barnsdall Ave

Hollywood Blvd

Sunset Blvd

Ⓜ **Vermont/
Sunset**

0   100   200   300 yards
0   100   200   300 meters

23 LOS FELIZ: WRIGHT'S ARCHITECTURAL GEMS AND SWINGERS' FAVORITE NIGHT SPOTS

BOUNDARIES: **Edgemont St., Glendower Ave., Hillhurst Ave., Sunset Blvd.**
THOMAS GUIDE COORDINATES: **Map 594; A3**
DISTANCE: **Approx. 1½ to 3½ miles (depending on route chosen)**
DIFFICULTY: **Strenuous (includes stairways)**
PARKING: **Free street parking is available on Catalina St.**
NEAREST METRO STATION: **Vermont Ave. and Sunset Blvd. (Red Line). Note: Change starting point of walk to Barnsdall Art Park if you take the Metro.**

Los Feliz, a charming, vibrant neighborhood just northeast of Hollywood, is fast becoming an exclusive address—particularly in the hills—and the rest of the region is quickly gentrifying as homebuyers come to appreciate the area's proximity to the wilderness of Griffith Park and the action of Hollywood and Silver Lake. Fans of Doug Liman's 1996 movie, *Swingers*, will recognize a couple of the night spots featured prominently in the film, the Dresden restaurant and bar and the Derby swing club, along Los Feliz's main drags.

This neighborhood is also notable for its architecture, in particular Frank Lloyd Wright's Ennis-Brown House, which is tucked high in the hills, and the architect's Hollyhock House, which sits just over a mile south in the flatlands. This route takes you into Los Feliz's affluent, hilly residential area before making an optional detour south through Los Feliz Village to Barnsdall Art Park, home of the Hollyhock House.

● **Begin at the corner of Los Feliz Blvd. and Catalina St. and head north on Catalina. The quiet, magnolia-lined street features attractive, expensive-looking homes. Look up to your left to see the Griffith Observatory, which appears surprisingly close in the hills above.**

● **Turn right on Cromwell Ave. and look for the Berendo stairway on your left, across the street from 2251 Berendo St.**

- Ascend the long stairway, which is shaded in places by overhanging oleander and bougainvillea bushes. About two thirds of the way up, you'll come to a landing with thoughtfully built-in benches.

- At the top of the stairs, turn right on Bonvue Ave. and follow the narrow road as it winds higher into the hills. Keep an eye out for cars around each sharp bend. This street has a very Mediterranean feel, with magnificent, two- and three-story Spanish homes built into the hill on the left.

- Eventually, you come to a split in the road. Continue straight on what is now Glendower Ave. You pass a Rudolf Schindler-designed home at 2567, but you can't see much of the building apart from the shimmering green outer wall. A few doors down, at 2587, is another eye-catching house; composed of metal and gray concrete, the industrial-looking structure towers over the road, supported by sturdy-looking cement columns. Finally, at 2607 Glendower, you reach the start of Frank Lloyd Wright's imposing and innovative Ennis-Brown House, one of several of the architect's textile block designs in the LA area. This massive structure, built in 1924, overlooks the Los Angeles basin below and is composed of cinder blocks carved with Mayan designs, giving it the look of an ancient fortress.

- Follow Glendower as it curves around the Ennis-Brown House, eventually lending a view of the north-facing façade of the home. The building is perhaps most recognizable as Harrison Ford's character's home in *Blade Runner*, although it's been featured in many other films. Continue west on Glendower. The eclectic architectural mix of homes on this high, sunny street boast spectacular views of the city below.

- Just before you reach 2763 Glendower, you'll see a signpost reading PUBLIC WALK. Descend these stairs down to Bryn Mawr Rd., pausing to admire the stunning vista of the hills to the northeast, and of the Ennis-Brown House to your left.

- Cross the cul-de-sac and continue down the next set of steps to Bonvue Ave. This stairway is enhanced by a colorful tiled mural that was funded by the Los Feliz neighbors association.

- At the bottom of the steps, cross the street to go straight on Glendower Ave. Follow the winding road past more beautiful homes as it gently leads downhill.

- Continue to follow the road as it curves sharply to the right, and avoid Glendower Pl., which branches off to the left.

- Glendower merges with Vermont Ave., which leads up to the Greek Theatre, a moderate-sized outdoor concert venue. Continue south on Vermont.

- At this point, you can either turn right on Los Feliz Blvd. and head a few blocks west to your starting point at Catalina St., or you can continue through Los Feliz Village to the Barnsdall Art Park, home of Frank Lloyd Wright's Hollyhock House. This optional addendum route is detailed below.

Addendum:

- Cross Los Feliz Blvd. and continue south on Vermont Ave. into Los Feliz Village. The first few blocks along Vermont consist mostly of apartment buildings and a few houses of worship. But after you cross Franklin Ave., it becomes more interesting. The thriving collection of shops and restaurants along the next few blocks includes the Electric Lotus Indian restaurant and adjacent Psychobabble coffeehouse; House of Pies, a middling family restaurant with a huge selection of doughy desserts; Palermo Italian Restaurant, where vino flows freely in the waiting lounge on busy nights; Fred 62, a retro diner for hipsters; the Los Feliz 3 movie theater; independent Skylight Books; Squaresville vintage clothing store;

Looking west from Barnsdall Art Park

the legendary Dresden Room; the classy Vermont Restaurant and Bar; and several more casual and upscale eateries, chic clothing shops, and home decor boutiques. It's amazing how many commercial points of interest are crammed into this short stretch of street.

- Turn right on Prospect Ave., which merges with Hollywood Blvd., to enter the Little Armenia neighborhood.

- Cross the street at New Hampshire Ave. and enter Barnsdall Art Park on the south side of Hollywood Blvd. This innovative community arts center sits atop Olive Hill and is virtually hidden from the streets below. In addition to the Los Angeles Municipal Arts Gallery and Junior Arts Center, the park is home to another Frank Lloyd Wright masterpiece, the Hollyhock House.

- Ascend the stairs into the park, turn right at the road (following the sign for the Gallery Theatre), and then ascend the next set of steps on your left to a beautiful, grassy park dotted with pine trees.

- If you'd like to learn more about the art programs at the park or pick up literature about the Hollyhock House, you can do so at the visitor's center on the left. Otherwise, continue straight along the path through the park, and then turn right

DESIGNER NAME: FRANK LLOYD WRIGHT

Born in 1867, Frank Lloyd Wright is probably America's best-known architect, renowned for masterpieces as diverse as the Guggenheim Museum in New York City and the Fallingwater residence in western Pennsylvania. Inspired by the wide-open prairies of his birthplace in Wisconsin, Wright introduced the idea of open floor plans and organic design in residential architecture.

In the early 1920s, Wright pioneered his concrete textile block style in Southern California. This innovative technique involved using pre-manufactured, engraved concrete blocks that were inset with glass to allow light to filter indoors. One advantage of this system was affordability, as concrete blocks made a cheap, modular building material. There are four examples of Wright's textile block architecture in the Los Angeles area—the Ennis-Brown House in Los Feliz, the Millard House in Pasadena, and the Samuel Freeman and John Storer houses in the Hollywood Hills.

to reach the Hollyhock House itself. This was Frank Lloyd Wright's first project in Los Angeles, pre-dating the Ennis-Brown House by several years. Wright used this project to create a regionally appropriate architectural style, which he referred to as "California Romanza." This style interweaves indoor and outdoor space, making extensive use of rooftop terraces and enclosed gardens.

- After exploring the park, retrace your steps to Hollywood Blvd.

- Cross the street at New Hampshire Ave. and turn right to retrace your steps along Prospect Ave.

- Cross Vermont Ave. and continue east on Prospect, passing several old wooden houses and a collection of slightly rundown apartment buildings.

- Turn left on Hillhurst Ave. This isn't exactly a pretty street, but it does feature numerous restaurants, bars, and coffeehouses that are popular with both locals and out-of-towners looking for an authentic "eastsider" experience. At 1760, you pass Home, a—you guessed it—*home*-style outdoor eatery that offers a few healthy twists on your traditional diner menu. At 1831, you encounter Ye Rustic Inn, a dive bar in a strip mall that has proven inexplicably popular with trend-seeking scenesters, as well as neighborhood drunks. Alcove Cafe & Bakery tempts passersby with a welcoming patio and a tantalizing array of baked goodies at 1929 Hillhurst.

  Near Los Feliz Blvd. are more food and drink venues: Mexico City, a decent, middle-price-range eatery that serves stiff margaritas; Tangiers

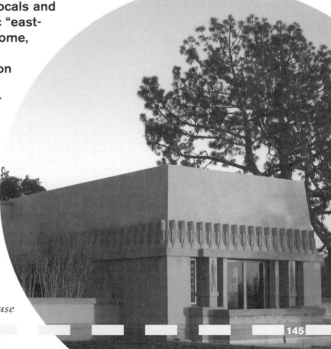

Frank Lloyd Wright's Hollyhock House

Lounge, a relatively new exotic hot spot; and, finally, the Derby, the swing-dancing club immortalized in *Swingers*, the film that provided a humorous glimpse into the nightlife of Hollywood's struggling actors on the brink of the late-'90s swing-dancing craze. For those interested in beauty and wellness, this stretch of Hillhurst also features an excellent yoga studio, Karuna Yoga, at 1939½ Hillhurst, and an intimate neighborhood spa, Being in LA, at 2016 Hillhurst.

● Turn left on Los Feliz Blvd. After you cross Vermont Ave., the homes on either side of the street become increasingly opulent. Continue for three more short blocks back to your starting point at the corner of Los Feliz and Catalina St.

POINTS OF INTEREST

Ennis-Brown House 2607 Glendower Ave., Los Angeles, CA 90027

Electric Lotus 4656 Franklin Ave., Los Angeles, CA 90027, 323-953-0040

Psychobabble 1866 N. Vermont Ave., Los Angeles, CA 90027, 323-664-7500

House of Pies 1869 N. Vermont Ave., Los Angeles, CA 90027, 323-666-9961

Palermo Italian Restaurant 1858 N. Vermont Ave., Los Angeles, CA 90027, 323-663-1178

Fred 62 1850 N. Vermont Ave., Los Angeles, CA 90027, 323-667-0062

Los Feliz 3 1822 N. Vermont Ave., Los Angeles, CA 90027, 323-664-2169

Skylight Books 1818 N. Vermont Ave., Los Angeles, CA 90027, 323-660-1175

Squaresville 1800 N. Vermont Ave., Los Angeles, CA 90027, 323-669-8464

Dresden Restaurant 1760 N. Vermont Ave., Hollywood, CA 90027, 323-665-4294

Vermont Restaurant and Bar 1714 N. Vermont Ave., Los Angeles, CA 90027, 323-661-6163

Barnsdall Art Park/Hollyhock House 4800 Hollywood Blvd., Los Angeles, CA 90027, 323-644-6269

Home 1760 Hillhurst Ave., Los Angeles, CA 90027, 323-669-0211

Alcove Cafe & Bakery 1929 Hillhurst Ave., Los Angeles, CA 90027, 323-644-0100

Mexico City 2121 Hillhurst Ave., Los Angeles, CA 90027, 323-661-7227

Tangiers Lounge 2138 Hillhurst Ave., Los Angeles, CA 90027, 323-666-8666

Derby 4500 Los Feliz Blvd., Los Angeles, CA 90027, 323-663-8979

Karuna Yoga 1939½ Hillhurst Ave., Los Angeles, CA 90027, 323-665-6242

Being in LA 2016 Hillhurst Ave., Los Angeles, CA 90027, 323-665-9355

route summary

1. Begin at the corner of Los Feliz Blvd. and Catalina St. and head north on Catalina.
2. Turn right on Cromwell Ave.
3. Ascend the stairway opposite 2251 Berendo St.
4. At the top of the stairs, turn right on Bonvue Ave.
5. Continue straight on Glendower Ave.
6. Follow Glendower as it curves around the Ennis-Brown House.
7. Descend the stairway next to 2763 Glendower.
8. Cross the cul-de-sac and continue down the next set of steps.
9. At the bottom of the steps, cross the street and continue straight on Glendower Ave.
10. Follow the road as it curves sharply to the right, and avoid Glendower Pl., which branches off to the left.
11. Glendower merges with Vermont Ave. Continue south on Vermont.
12. Turn right on Los Feliz Blvd. to return to your starting point at Catalina St., or continue on the following optional addendum.

Addendum:

13. Cross Los Feliz Blvd. and continue south on Vermont Ave.
14. Turn right on Prospect Ave., which merges with Hollywood Blvd.
15. Cross the street at New Hampshire Ave. and enter Barnsdall Art Park on the south side of Hollywood Blvd.
16. Ascend the stairs into the park, turn right at the road, and then ascend the next set of steps on your left.
17. Continue straight along the path through the park, and then turn right to reach the Hollyhock House.
18. Retrace your steps to Hollywood Blvd.
19. Cross the street at New Hampshire and turn right to retrace your steps along Prospect Ave.
20. Cross Vermont Ave. and continue east on Prospect.
21. Turn left on Hillhurst Ave.
22. Turn left on Los Feliz Blvd. and walk several blocks back to your starting point at Catalina St.

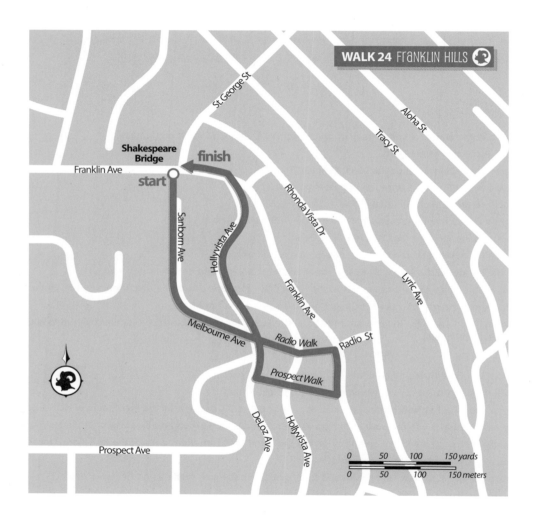

St. George St

Aloha St

Tracy St

Shakespeare
Bridge

finish

Franklin Ave

start

Rhonda Vista Dr

Sanborn Ave

Hollyvista Ave

Franklin Ave

Lyric Ave

Melbourne Ave

Radio Walk

Radio St

Prospect Walk

DeLoz Ave

Hollyvista Ave

Prospect Ave

0 50 100 150 yards
0 50 100 150 meters

24 FranKLIN HILLS:
WHAT LIES ON THE OTHER SIDE OF THE BRIDGE

BOUNDARIES: **Franklin Ave., Fountain Ave., Talmadge St., Hyperion Ave.**
THOMAS GUIDE COORDINATES: **Map 594; B3**
DISTANCE: **Approx. ½ mile**
DIFFICULTY: **Moderate (includes stairways)**
PARKING: **Free street parking is available on the north side of Franklin Ave., east of the Shakespeare Bridge.**

Nestled between Los Feliz and Silver Lake, Franklin Hills is another of central Los Angeles' endearing hilly neighborhoods. This residential area was developed in the 1920s as a quiet community centrally located in the midst of the sprawling metro area, and today it retains an old-fashioned, neighborly quality that many of LA's newer developments lack. This impression is reinforced by the two very long concrete stairways that connect the region's winding streets, giving neighbors relatively easy walking access to one another's homes, while at the same time keeping their hearts and lungs in great condition.

● Begin just east of the Shakespeare Bridge on Franklin Ave. The distinctive white structure was built in 1926 and bridged the way, so to speak, for the charming residential neighborhood of Franklin Hills. Walk to the south side of the street, just past the house that sits immediately east of the bridge, and descend the ficus- and bougainvillea-shaded staircase leading down just beyond the sign for St. George St.

● You emerge in the cul-de-sac at the north end of Sanborn Ave. Continue south on Sanborn; most of the homes on this street are simple and modern in design, and a few are painted in vibrant colors. On your right, pass a community garden with a variety of vegetables that was planted by the people living here. Behind the garden is a community picnic area and playground.

● Follow the road as it curves to the left and becomes Melbourne Ave. Most of the homes here are modest, well maintained, and exhibit a variety of architectural styles—traditional, Spanish Colonial Revival, and English country cottage. The Spanish-style home at 3916 Melbourne is especially lovely, with cheerful yellow paint, gorgeous tile work, and an elegant fountain in the front yard. Next door, at 3912, is a dramatically different style of home—a fairytale English cottage with a deeply sloping wood-shingled roof and diamond-pane windows.

- Continue straight across DeLoz Ave. and look for the sign for the Radio Walk steps just to the right of 1856 DeLoz. Ascend the long staircase, which is overgrown with a thick layer of dead leaves, giving it the feel of a secret passage. Cross Hollyvista Ave. and continue up the next flight of steps, which is more heavily shaded than the first half of Radio Walk.

- Emerge on Franklin Ave., just north of Radio St. Turn right to cross Radio St. and continue on Franklin. You can catch occasional glimpses of the Griffith Observatory between the houses on your right.

- Turn right just past 3818 Franklin to descend the Prospect Walk stairway, and pause at the top of steps to admire the view east along Hollywood Blvd., which stretches out below. Cross Hollyvista Ave. and continue down the next set of steps.

- When you reach DeLoz Ave., turn right instead of descending the last flight of Prospect Walk stairs. DeLoz is a quiet, sunny street with lots of cute, Spanish-style houses, French and English cottages, and many traditional homes. The houses built into the steeply sloping hill on the right appear to be much larger than those on the left side of the street, but appearances can be deceiving with these hillside homes.

- Cross Prospect Ave. and continue on DeLoz Ave., passing the Radio Walk steps you ascended earlier. This is a bit of a tricky intersection, as it marks the connection of DeLoz, Prospect, and Melbourne, so be sure to continue straight ahead on your path, rather than wandering off on one of these offshoots.

- DeLoz Ave. ends when it merges with Hollyvista Ave. Continue straight on what is now Hollyvista. At 2024, take note of a delightful home with blue awnings, a wood-shingled roof, and a white picket fence—the picture of blissful domesticity. A large, austere, modern home sits in stark contrast at 2100 Hollyvista.

● **Turn left at the next intersection to head west on Franklin Ave., and you will shortly return to your starting point just east of the Shakespeare Bridge.**

route summary

1. Begin just east of the Shakespeare Bridge on Franklin Ave. Descend the stairway on the south side of the street next to the street sign for St. George St.
2. Emerge on the cul-de-sac at the north end of Sanborn Ave. and continue south on Sanborn.
3. Follow the road as it curves to the left, becoming Melbourne Ave.
4. Continue straight across DeLoz Ave. and ascend the Radio Walk steps just to the right of 1856 DeLoz.
5. Cross Hollyvista Ave. and continue up the next flight of steps.
6. Emerge on Franklin Ave., just north of Radio St., and turn right to cross Radio St. and continue on Franklin.
7. Turn right just past 3818 Franklin to descend the Prospect Walk stairway.
8. Cross Hollyvista Ave. and continue down the next set of steps.
9. When you reach DeLoz Ave., turn right instead of descending the last flight of Prospect Walk stairs.
10. Where DeLoz Ave. ends, continue straight on what is now Hollyvista Ave.
11. Turn left at Franklin Ave. to return to your starting point just east of the Shakespeare Bridge.

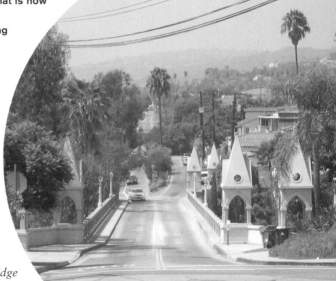

Shakespeare Bridge

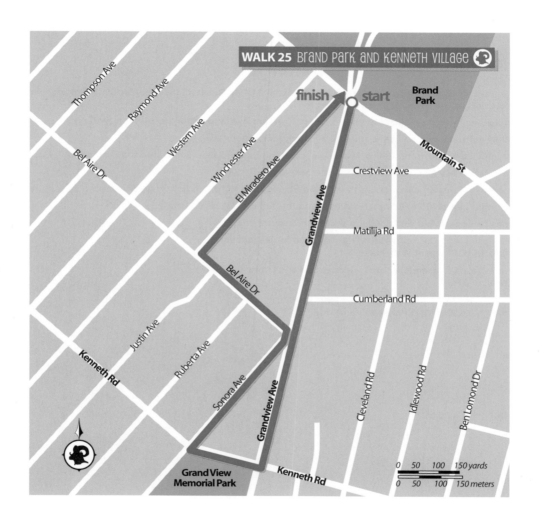

finish   start

Brand Park

Thompson Ave

Raymond Ave

Western Ave

Winchester Ave

Bel Aire Dr

El Miradero Ave

Grandview Ave

Mountain St

Crestview Ave

Matilija Rd

Cumberland Rd

Bel Aire Dr

Justin Ave

Ruberta Ave

Sonora Ave

Kenneth Rd

Grandview Ave

Kenneth Rd

Cleveland Rd

Idlewood Rd

Ben Lomond Dr

Grand View
Memorial Park

0   50   100   150 yards
0   50   100   150 meters

25 BranD park anD kenneth village: GlenDale turns on the charm

BOUNDARIES: Brand Park, Grandview Ave., Kenneth Rd., Western Ave.
THOMAS GUIDE COORDINATES: Map 534; B7
DISTANCE: Approx. 1½ miles
DIFFICULTY: Moderate
PARKING: Free parking is available in the Brand Park parking lot.

Located between Burbank and Pasadena, the city of Glendale bridges the gap between the San Fernando and San Gabriel valleys. This walk explores two of Glendale's more charming attractions, Brand Park and Kenneth Village. The Brand Library & Art Center, located inside Brand Park, was built in 1904 as the home of Leslie Coombs Brand, an early developer in the Glendale area. He named his mansion "El Miradero," and a gateway bearing this name still stands at the entrance to the park. After exploring the park, you'll head downhill to Kenneth Village, which lends a delightful small-town character to this part of Glendale.

- Begin in Brand Park, at the intersection of Mountain St. and Grandview Ave., where you can spend some time exploring the park and the Brand Library & Art Center. The unique and lovely structure combines element of Spanish, Moorish, and Indian architecture. Stop in to peruse the library's impressive art and music collections or to admire the latest exhibition in the adjacent gallery. While in the park, you may also want to visit the Whispering Pine Treehouse & Friendship Garden, a lovely little Japanese garden and pond, as well as the Victorian Doctor's House Museum and Gazebo. The Doctor's House was the former residence of three prominent Glendale physicians and has been restored to its late 19th century appearance.

- Exit the park onto Grandview Ave. A grand villa catches the eye to your left, at 1770 Mountain St. Head south on Grandview, going slightly downhill away from Brand Park. The street is lined with beautifully maintained homes, and the neighborhood gives the impression of being friendly and family oriented—you may see several mothers (or nannies) out with strollers. Use caution walking on Grandview, however, as the sidewalk stops and starts, and this is a fairly high-trafficked street.

- Turn right on Kenneth Rd. You're now in the midst of Kenneth Village, Glendale's diminutive, old-fashioned downtown area. This one-block stretch has a pleasing small-town vibe and is home to a neighborhood pharmacy, meat market, salons, and a florist. A couple of notable shops include Retro Parc, a vintage home-furnishings store and Audrey K., which sells some very cute women's clothing and accessories. Many of the stores on this street keep odd hours—Monday, for example, is not a good day to shop on Kenneth Rd. Take your time strolling the street: Treat yourself to a pastry at Village French Bakery, stop to admire the puppies in the window at Pet Rush, or pick up a bouquet at Ivy's Flower Station, which is housed in a quaint former gas station at the corner of Kenneth and Sonora Ave.

- Turn right on Sonora. Enjoy the view of the foothills and mountains ahead as you stroll slightly uphill along this residential street. The neighborhood features an eclectic architectural mix—Mediterranean, Norman, Cape Cod, and traditional—and most of the homes have broad green lawns.

- Turn left on Bel Aire Dr. This street's residences range in style and size; modest traditional homes stand alongside grand Mediterranean villas. The large wood-shingled house with a steeply pitched roof and stone chimney catches the eye at 1600 Bel Aire.

- Turn right on El Miradero Ave. The architecture here is remarkably cohesive, consisting mostly of meticulously maintained Spanish-style homes, many with distinctive flourishes such as colorful tilework and arched picture windows. As you near the end of El Miradero at Mountain St., you'll see the white Brand Park entrance gate ahead.

- Walk through the gate to return to your starting point inside Brand Park.

POINTS OF INTEREST

Brand Library & Art Center 1601 West Mountain St., Glendale, CA 91201, 818-548-2051

Retro Parc 1405 W Kenneth Rd., Glendale, CA 91201, 818-242-3104

Audrey K. 1411½ W. Kenneth Rd., Glendale, CA 91201, 818-242-5758

Village French Bakery 1414 W. Kenneth Rd. Glendale, CA 91201, 818-241-2521

Pet Rush 1420 W. Kenneth Rd. Glendale, CA 91201, 818-956-0029

Ivy's Flower Station 1435 W. Kenneth Rd., Glendale, CA 91201, 818-500-7599

ROUTE SUMMARY

1. Begin in Brand Park, at the intersection of Mountain St. and Grandview Ave., and spend some time exploring the park.
2. Exit the park onto Grandview Ave. and head south.
3. Turn right on Kenneth Rd.
4. Turn right on Sonora Ave.
5. Turn left on Bel Aire Dr.
6. Turn right on El Miradero Ave.
7. Return to your starting point inside Brand Park.

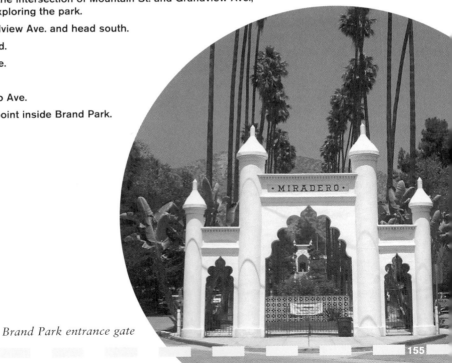

Brand Park entrance gate

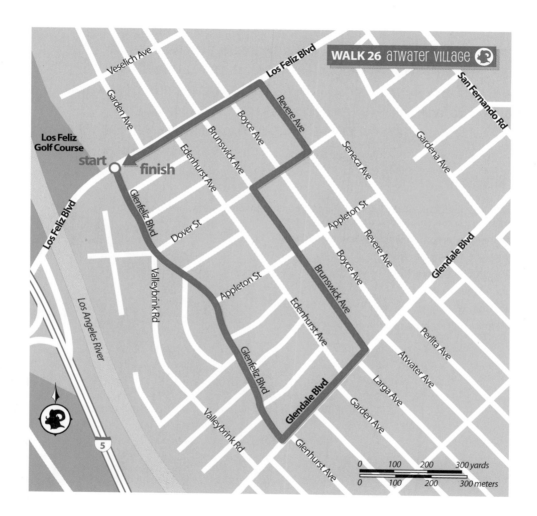

Veselich Ave

Los Feliz Blvd

San Fernando Rd

Garden Ave

Los Feliz
Golf Course

start

finish

Boyce Ave

Revere Ave

Brunswick Ave

Edenhurst Ave

Gardena Ave

Seneca Ave

Los Feliz Blvd

Glenfeliz Blvd

Dover St

Appleton St

Revere Ave

Glendale Blvd

Valleybrink Rd

Appleton St

Boyce Ave

Brunswick Ave

Los Angeles River

Glenfeliz Blvd

Edenhurst Ave

Perlita Ave

Atwater Ave

Valleybrink Rd

Glendale Blvd

Larga Ave

Garden Ave

5

Glenhurst Ave

| 0 | 100 | 200 | 300 yards |
| 0 | 100 | 200 | 300 meters |

26 atwater village: a hipster's haven

BOUNDARIES: **Los Feliz Blvd., 5 Freeway, Glendale Blvd., San Fernando Rd.**
THOMAS GUIDE COORDINATES: **Map 594; D1**
DISTANCE: **Approx. 2 miles**
DIFFICULTY: **Easy**
PARKING: **Free street parking is available on Glenfeliz Blvd.**

Sandwiched between Los Feliz and Glendale, Atwater Village offers charming residential neighborhoods as well as a burgeoning dining and shopping scene. The neighborhood has long been home to low-key watering holes like the Roost and Bigfoot Lodge, which attract hipsters from nearby Hollywood, Silver Lake, and Los Feliz. And the opening of an upscale day spa and a handful of trendy shops and restaurants are only going to add to the appeal of this formerly under-the-radar 'hood.

- Begin at the corner of Glenfeliz Blvd. and Los Feliz Blvd. and head south on Glenfeliz, passing an elementary school on your left as you head away from busy Los Feliz Blvd. into a relatively quiet residential neighborhood.

- After crossing Dover St., bear left to remain on Glenfeliz. The street is lined with shady sycamore trees and features quaint, modest-sized homes in a predominantly Spanish architectural style.

- Turn left on Glendale Blvd. This stretch of the busy thoroughfare is home to a variety of small businesses; the mix includes everything from dentists and insurance offices to upscale home furnishings and pet boutiques. Thankfully, there are also some good dining options here. Indochine Vien, at 3110, serves up mouthwatering pho and other affordable Vietnamese tasties, while Tacos Villa Corona, at 3185, is the spot for what very well may be the best potato tacos you've ever tasted (for just a buck!). And if you're in the mood for some retro flavor, stop in at Club Tee Gee, at 3210, which has been around since 1946 and has the decor to match (re-created after a fire destroyed the interior in 1993).

- Turn left on Brunswick Ave. Notice the colorful "fantasy bungalows" at 3642 and 3648. These 1920s-built homes combine Egyptian and Norman architectural styles to unique and whimsical effect, and are so named because their style shows the influence of silent movie sets from that period. At 3742 is another notable home featuring trapezoidal windows. Apart from these standouts, the street is home to a hodgepodge of residential architecture, featuring mainly Craftsman and Mediterranean homes.

- Turn right on Dover St. and walk for two short blocks to Revere Ave.

- Turn left on Revere.

- Turn left on Los Feliz Blvd. Straight ahead is a large shopping complex featuring a Costco, Toys "R" Us, Best Buy, and various chain restaurants. At 2980 is the Tudor-style Tam O'Shanter Inn, part of the venerable Lawry's restaurant family that specializes in prime rib. Inside, waitresses dressed in Scottish tartan serve up tasty fare such as Yorkshire pudding, Toad in the Hole, and, of course, prime rib. While the atmosphere is a bit stuffy and the prices steep, dining here is a unique experience, and the food is undeniably delicious.

  Other notable locations on this stretch of Los Feliz Blvd. include neighborhood watering holes the Roost and Bigfoot Lodge, at 3100 and 3172, respectively; India Sweets and Spices, which features a casual cafeteria where you can snack on tasty vegetarian Indian fare or enjoy a complete meal on the cheap, at 3126; and Potted, a fun and eclectic garden design shop, at 3158. On the north side of the street are the LA Bread bakery and cafe, at 3119; Asia, an upscale Cal-Asian eatery, at 3179; and the Los Feliz Municipal Golf Course, an affordable nine-hole course tucked into the corner of Griffith Park, at 3207 Los Feliz Blvd. (You may choose to forgo the links and enjoy a greasy bite at an outdoor table at the course's Los Feliz Cafe.)

- Return to your starting point at the corner of Glenfeliz Blvd. To reward yourself for your nearly 2-mile trek, consider dropping in at dtox Day Spa (just past Glenfeliz at 3206 Los Feliz Blvd.). This pampering sanctuary is housed in a beautifully converted industrial space and offers Zen-inspired treatments and all the spa amenities you need to unwind completely.

POINTS OF INTEREST

Indochine Vien 3110 Glendale Blvd., Los Angeles, CA 90039, 323-667-9591

Tacos Villa Corona 3185 Glendale Blvd., Los Angeles, CA 90039, 323-661-3458

Club Tee Gee 3210 Glendale Blvd., Los Angeles, CA 90039, 323-669-9631

Tam O'Shanter Inn 2980 Los Feliz Blvd., Los Angeles, CA 90039, 323-664-0228

Roost 3100 Los Feliz Blvd., Los Angeles, CA 90039, 323-664-7272

Bigfoot Lodge 3172 Los Feliz Blvd., Los Angeles, CA 90039, 323-662-9227

India Sweets and Spices 3126 Los Feliz Blvd., Los Angeles, CA 90039, 323-345-0360

Potted 3158 Los Feliz Blvd., Los Angeles, CA 90039, 323-665-3801

LA Bread 3119 Los Feliz Blvd., Los Angeles, CA 90039, 323-662-8600

Asia 3179 Los Feliz Blvd., Los Angeles, CA 90039, 323-906-9498

Los Feliz Municipal Golf Course 3207 Los Feliz Blvd.,
Los Angeles, CA 90039, 323-663-7758

dtox Day Spa 3206 Los Feliz Blvd., Los Angeles, CA
90039, 323-665-3869

ROUTE SUMMARY

1. Begin at the corner of Glenfeliz Blvd. and Los Feliz Blvd. and head south on Glenfeliz.
2. After crossing Dover St., bear left to remain on Glenfeliz.
3. Turn left on Glendale Blvd.
4. Turn left on Brunswick Ave.
5. Turn right on Dover St.
6. Turn left on Revere Ave.
7. Turn left on Los Feliz Blvd.
8. Return to your starting point at the corner of Glenfeliz Blvd.

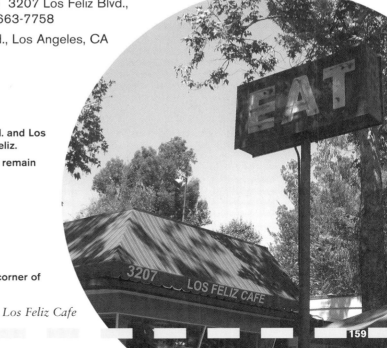

Los Feliz Cafe

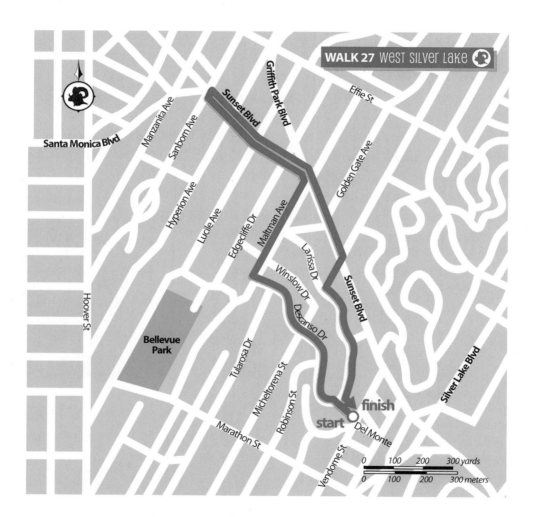

WALK 27 WEST SILVER LAKE

Effie St

Griffith Park Blvd

Golden Gate Ave

Sunset Blvd

Santa Monica Blvd

Manzanita Ave

Sanborn Ave

Hyperion Ave

Lucile Ave

Edgecliffe Dr

Maltman Ave

Larissa Dr

Winslow Dr

Descanso Dr

Sunset Blvd

Silver Lake Blvd

Hoover St

Bellevue
Park

Tularosa Dr

Micheltorena St

Robinson St

Marathon St

Vendome St

start

finish

Del Monte

0 100 200 300 yards

0 100 200 300 meters

27 WeST SILVeR Lake: SUNSeT JUNCTION, WHaT'S YOUR FUNCTION?

BOUNDARIES: Sunset Blvd., Silver Lake Blvd., Marathon St., Hoover St.
THOMAS GUIDE COORDINATES: Map 594; C6
DISTANCE: Approx. 1¾ miles
DIFFICULTY: Moderate (includes stairways)
PARKING: Free street parking is available on Vendome St.

Every summer, the Sunset Junction Neighborhood Alliance puts on a street fair at the intersection of Sunset and Santa Monica boulevards that perfectly illustrates the unique dichotomy of Silver Lake: The huge event celebrates the area's diversity, as the predominantly white rockers, hipsters, and scruffy artists who have flocked to the area in recent years, and the Mexican-American families who have lived here for generations, come to party. Even if you can't make the street fair—which typically features performances by local bands and an endless variety of vendors hawking clothing, jewelry, incense, and, of course, lots of great stuff to eat—this is a great neighborhood to visit. This walk explores the area's residential streets, as well as the main commercial drag along Sunset Blvd., which features a cool and eclectic collections of shops, restaurants, and cafes.

● Begin at the intersection of Vendome St. and Del Monte Dr., just south of Sunset Blvd. On the west side of Vendome, across from the intersection of Del Monte, are the famous Music Box Steps, immortalized in Laurel and Hardy's 1932 short film, *The Music Box*, in which the duo attempted to move a piano up the 133 steps and hilarity ensued.

● Ascend the staircase to Descanso Dr., climb another short flight of steps to the second level of the split street, and then turn left.

● Follow Descanso Dr. as it curves to the right. On the northwest corner of Descanso Dr. and Micheltorena St. is a cheerful home painted with sunflowers; the front gate is decorated with a mosaic angel. Continue on Descanso across Micheltorena, and notice how the homes become more attractively maintained as you head farther up the hill.

- When you reach the end of Descanso Dr., turn right on Maltman Ave. Follow the road over the crest of the hill, and then all the way down to Sunset Blvd.

- Turn left on Sunset. On the opposite side of the street are El Conquistador, a vibrant Mexican restaurant that serves up a mean margarita, Pazzo Gelato, Good Microbrew and Grill, and other tempting dining options.

Once you cross Lucile Ave., the abundance of funky specialty shops is a sure sign of this neighborhood's uniquely hip style of gentrification. Trendy home furnishings stores line the northeast side of Sunset, while the southwest side features an eclectic array of shops and cafes. Upscale gift shops and baby boutiques sit next door to vintage clothing stores and the Surplus Value Center, where you can stock up on Dickies gear and fatigues. Clever names like Den of Antiquity, Pull My Daisy, and Eat Well signal the creativity of Silver Lake's small business owners.

As you approach Sanborn Ave., note the Sunset Junction sign over the sidewalk. Intelligentsia, a gourmet and eco-friendly coffeehouse holds court at 3922 Sunset. The cluster of shops on the corner, several of which are hidden from the street, includes the Cheese Store of Silver Lake and a flower shop. Lovecraft Biofuels is just across Sanborn, at 4000 Sunset. This innovative auto shop can covert any diesel engine to run on vegetable oil.

- Turn around at Sanborn Ave. to retrace your steps back to Maltman Ave. Cross Maltman and continue along Sunset Blvd., passing the charming Madame Matisse cafe on the corner, and Millie's, a no-frills diner frequented by the neighborhood's edgier artists and rockers, located at 3524. The strip mall next door is home to Alegria on Sunset, whose unassuming exterior belies the vibrant atmosphere within—this is an excellent spot for *aguas frescas* and authentic Mexican specialties drenched in mole sauce.

- When you reach Micheltorena St., look for the short sidewalk that leads to a long stairway on your right; an interesting wooden rotunda sits in the enclosed yard to the left of the sidewalk. Ascend the Micheltorena steps as far as Larissa Dr. and turn left (don't climb the second flight of steps).

- Continue along Larissa, keeping to the right when the road splits, at which point it becomes Descanso Dr.

- Follow Descanso Dr. uphill, and keep an eye out for the short flight of steps that cuts across the meridian on your left.

- Descend these steps and then cross to the other side of the street, back to the Music Box Steps, which you climbed earlier. Head downstairs to return to your starting point on Vendome St.

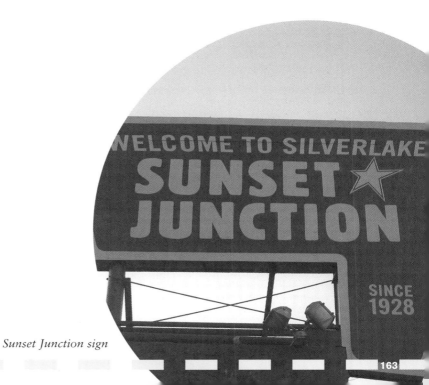

Sunset Junction sign

POINTS OF INTEREST

El Conquistador 3701 W. Sunset Blvd., Los Angeles, CA 90026, 323-666-0265
Pazzo Gelato 3827 W. Sunset Blvd., Los Angeles, CA 90026, 323-662-1710
Good Microbrew and Grill 3725 W. Sunset Blvd., Los Angeles, CA 90029, 323-660-3645
Surplus Value Center 3828 W. Sunset Blvd., Los Angeles, CA 90026, 323-662-8132
Den of Antiquity 3902 W. Sunset Blvd., Los Angeles, CA 90029, 323-666-3881
Pull My Daisy 3908 W. Sunset Blvd., Los Angeles, CA 90029, 323-663-0608
Eat Well 3916 W. Sunset Blvd., Los Angeles, CA 90029, 323-664-1624
Intelligentsia Coffee and Tea 3922 W. Sunset Blvd., Los Angeles, CA 90026, 323-663-6173
Cheese Store of Silver Lake 3926 W. Sunset Blvd., Los Angeles, CA 90029, 323-644-7511
Lovecraft Biofuels 4000 W. Sunset Blvd., Los Angeles, CA 90029, 323-644-9072
Madame Matisse 3536 W. Sunset Blvd., Los Angeles, CA 90026, 323-662-4862
Millie's 3524 W. Sunset Blvd., Los Angeles, CA 90026, 323-664-0404
Alegria on Sunset 3510 W. Sunset Blvd., Los Angeles, CA 90026, 323-913-1422

route summary

1. Begin at the intersection of Vendome St. and Del Monte Dr., just south of Sunset Blvd.
2. Ascend the staircase on the west side of Vendome to Descanso Dr., climb another short flight of steps up to the second level of the split street, and then turn left.
3. Follow Descanso Dr. as it curves around to the right.
4. Turn right on Maltman Ave.
5. Turn left on Sunset Blvd.
6. Turn around at Sanborn Ave. and retrace your steps on Sunset to Maltman Ave.
7. Cross Maltman and continue on Sunset Blvd.
8. Turn right at Micheltorena St., following the sidewalk that leads to the long stairway.
9. Ascend the Micheltorena steps as far as Larissa Dr. and turn left (don't climb the second flight of steps).
10. Continue on Larissa, keeping to the right when the road splits, at which point it becomes Descanso Dr.
11. Follow Descanso Dr. uphill, keeping an eye out for the short flight of steps that cuts across the meridian on your left.
12. Descend the stairs and cross the street to reach the Music Box Steps, then head back downstairs to return to your starting point on Vendome St.

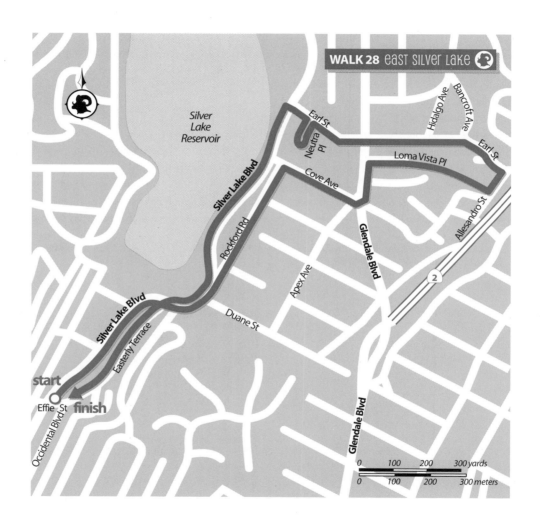

WALK 28 east silver lake

Silver
Lake
Reservoir

Earl St

Hidalgo Ave

Bancroft Ave

Earl St

Neutra Pl

Loma Vista Pl

Silver Lake Blvd

Cove Ave

Rockford Rd

Glendale Blvd

Allesandro St

2

Apex Ave

Silver Lake Blvd

Duane St

Easterly Terrace

start

finish

Effie St

Occidental Blvd

Glendale Blvd

| 0 | 100 | 200 | 300 yards |
| 0 | 100 | 200 | 300 meters |

28 east silver Lake: Modern Masterpieces above sparkling waters

BOUNDARIES: **Silver Lake Blvd., Glendale Blvd., 2 Freeway, Earl St.**
THOMAS GUIDE COORDINATES: **Map 594; D6**
DISTANCE: **Approx. 2 miles**
DIFFICULTY: **Strenuous (includes stairways)**
PARKING: **Free street parking is available on Silver Lake Blvd.**

Silver Lake is a popular destination for Los Angeles' gay, artist, and musician communities, as well as for culturally diverse young families who have found that the neighborhood's picturesque hills and lively community spirit make it a desirable alternative to more cost-prohibitive areas like the West Side or the Hollywood Hills. This route starts in one of the neighborhood's destinations for daytime shopping and nighttime music, and then climbs into the hills overlooking the Silver Lake Reservoir, where you'll discover rustic, overgrown walkways and homes that seem so far removed from LA's urban sprawl, you'll hardly believe you're only a few minutes from downtown.

● **Begin on Silver Lake Blvd. near the intersection with Effie St., and head northeast. For the most part, Silver Lake Blvd. is lined with houses and apartment buildings, but this short stretch features a collection of cute stores and cafes. At Yolk (1626 Silver Lake Blvd.), you can choose from a selection of uniquely hip merchandise such as children's toys, home decorations, architectural books, and yummy-scented candles. Across the street is an elegant interior design firm ironically called Rubbish. Neighborhood pizzeria Michelangelo is located a couple of doors down, at 1637 Silver Lake Blvd.**

At 1710, you come to the Back Door Bakery and Cafe, a casual breakfast and lunch spot with an outdoor patio popular with locals and their dogs. Spaceland, Silver Lake's main venue for live music from about-to-break bands, resides at 1717 Silver Lake Blvd. After crossing Van Pelt Pl., you'll see where all of the dogs at Back Door came from—the Silver Lake Recreation Center and off-leash dog park sits at the base

of the neighborhood's namesake reservoir, on the east side of the street. At 1886 Silver Lake Blvd. is a fairytale-like Tudor Revival house.

- After crossing Duane St., you come to a fork in the road where Rockford Rd. splits off from Silver Lake Blvd. to the right. Follow Rockford uphill. At 1948 Rockford is a striking modern home with a shallow, peaked roof and jutting eaves over the garage that give the structure a top-heavy look. Next door is a mysterious, gated compound with a long stairway that presumably leads up to Apex Ave., which runs parallel to Rockford. You can catch occasional glimpses down to the sparkling blue reservoir between the houses on your left.

- Turn right on Cove Ave. Look for the wide stairway up ahead and ascend its shallow steps, stopping to turn and admire the spectacular vista of the reservoir, the hills of Silver Lake, and, in the distance, the Hollywood sign and the dome of Griffith Park observatory. The homes on either side of the stairway are concealed by lush vegetation—palm trees, ivy, and succulents.

- At the top of the stairs, continue straight on Cove for one more block to Apex Ave., and turn left, following it down the hill toward Glendale Blvd. Despite the picturesque surroundings, some of the homes in this neighborhood are unkempt, with peeling paint and messy yards.

- At the diagonal intersection of Apex Ave. and Glendale Blvd., *carefully* cross Glendale (there is no crosswalk) and then turn left to head north on Glendale.

- Turn right on Loma Vista Pl. At 2384, look for the whimsical house with wavy walls and colorful mosaics that bring to mind the architecture of Antonio Gaudi.

- Ascend the steps at the end of the cul-de-sac. This combination stairway and walkway may well be the longest one in Los Angeles. Heavily overgrown in places and lined on either side with bungalows and farmhouses, the Loma Vista Pl. path has a distinctly rural feel. Eventually, the shady staircase widens and starts to head downhill. At this point, you can hear the dull roar of the 2 Freeway just ahead, startling you back into awareness of your urban surroundings.

- When you reach the end of the Loma Vista Pl. stairs, turn left on Allesandro St., which runs right next to the freeway. Across the freeway, you can see the hills of Elysian Park, LA's second largest urban wilderness, after Griffith Park.

- Turn left on Earl St. and bear right to avoid Earl Ct.

- When you reach the intersection of Earl St. and Bancroft Ave., look for a stairway near the street sign. Ascend the Earl St. steps, an extensive, zigzagging stairway.

- At the top of the stairs, continue straight on Earl St., which heads downhill at a sharp angle after it crosses Hidalgo Ave. As you descend the hill toward Glendale Blvd., the reservoir comes into view once more. Many of the homes are elevated above the street and concealed behind dense thickets of trees and ivy; the residents obviously value their privacy.

- Once again, *carefully* cross Glendale Blvd. and continue on Earl St. This stretch of Earl features several architecturally interesting houses. At 2425 is a lovely Spanish home with vibrant blue trim and a mailbox covered in brightly colored tile. At 2434 Earl St., you'll notice a stepped structure covered in weathered wood shingles. This is the Treetops triplex, which was designed in 1980 by Dion Neutra, son of acclaimed modernist architect Richard Neutra. Next door, at the corner of Earl St. and Neutra Pl., shrouded by bamboo and trees, is the headquarters of the Institute for Survival Through Design, run by Dion Neutra himself.

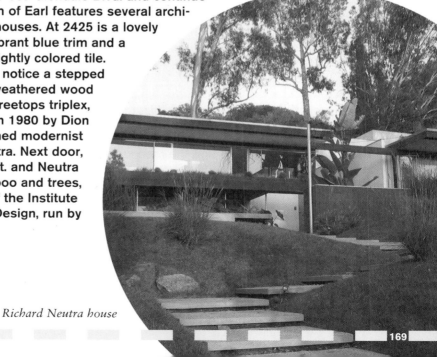

Richard Neutra house

- Turn left on Neutra Pl. This short cul-de-sac is a showcase of the architecture of Dion's father, famed first-generation modernist architect Richard Neutra. You can see examples of his work at 2218, 2200, and 2210 Neutra Pl. The O'Hara House, at 2210, is particularly striking; perched high above the street to afford views of the reservoir through its giant picture windows, the structure is a study of geometric shapes in glass and wood.

- Retrace your steps to Earl St. and turn left toward Silver Lake Blvd.

- Turn left on Silver Lake Blvd. You're now level with the reservoir just across the street. This stretch of the boulevard is rather pleasant, shaded with towering pines and eucalyptus trees. As you head south on Silver Lake, you pass another string of Richard Neutra-designed homes on your left, from 2226 to 2238 Silver Lake Blvd.

- Continue to walk alongside the reservoir for just under a half mile. After crossing Rockford St., retrace your steps from earlier for a couple of short blocks before turning left on Easterly Terrace and leaving the noisy boulevard behind. Easterly Terrace is an elevated residential street that runs roughly parallel to Silver Lake

DESIGNER NAME: RICHARD NEUTRA

Born in Vienna in 1892, Richard Neutra came to be one of the leaders of the Southern California modern architecture movement. After training with Otto Wagner in Austria, Neutra was drawn to the United States by American architectural legend Frank Lloyd Wright, and he eventually settled in California, where he worked closely with another Viennese-born Modernist icon, Rudolph Schindler. Neutra's signature designs consist of a light metal frame with a stucco or wood finish and extensive use of glass, creating an effect that manages to be both light and industrial. His buildings also take advantage of the region's amenable climate by carefully integrating residential landscapes into the structural design.

Neutra found Silver Lake to be LA's most open-minded neighborhood in terms of innovative architecture, so he built his home and studio in the hills overlooking the reservoir, and he also designed several more houses in this neighborhood.

Blvd. Large homes sit high above on the steep hill to your left, some teetering on stilts.

- When you reach the fork in the road at Occidental Blvd., go right to head downhill on Occidental.

- Turn right on Effie St. There's no sign, but it's the first cross street you come to on Occidental Blvd.

- Follow Effie for one short block to your starting point at Silver Lake Blvd.

POINTS OF INTEREST

Yolk 1626 Silver Lake Blvd., Los Angeles, CA 90026, 323-660-4315

Rubbish 1627 Silver Lake Blvd., Los Angeles, CA 90026, 323-661-5575

Michelangelo Pizzeria Ristorante 1637 Silver Lake Blvd., Los Angeles, CA 90026, 323-660-4843

Back Door Bakery and Cafe 1710 Silver Lake Blvd., Los Angeles, CA 90026, 323-662-7927

Spaceland 1717 Silver Lake Blvd., Los Angeles, CA 90026, 323-662-7728

Silver Lake Recreation Center 1850 Silver Lake Blvd., Los Angeles, CA 90026, 323-644-3946

route summary

1. Begin at the intersection of Silver Lake Blvd. and Effie St. and head north on Silver Lake.
2. Bear right on Rockford Rd.
3. Turn right on Cove Ave. and ascend the stairway.
4. Turn left on Apex Ave.
5. Turn left on Glendale Blvd.
6. Turn right on Loma Vista Pl.
7. Ascend the stairway/walkway and follow it back downhill.
8. Turn left on Allesandro St.
9. Turn left on Earl St. and bear right to avoid Earl Ct.
10. Ascend the stairs at the intersection with Bancroft Ave.
11. At the top of the stairs, continue on Earl St.
12. Turn left on Neutra Pl.
13. Return to Earl St. and turn left.
14. Turn left on Silver Lake Blvd.
15. Turn left on Easterly Terrace.
16. Bear right on Occidental Blvd.
17. Turn right on Effie St. to return to your starting point at the intersection of Effie and Silver Lake Blvd.

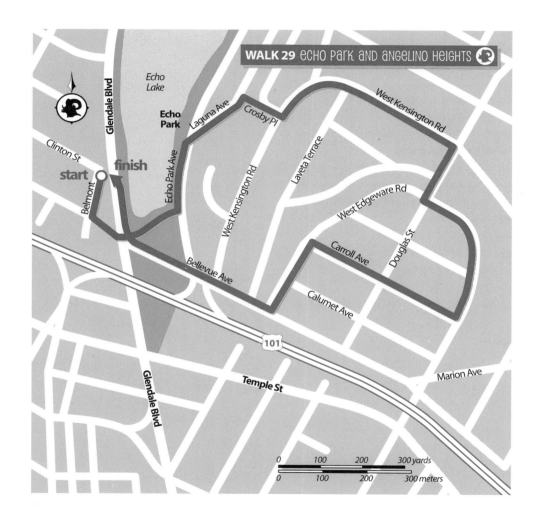

Echo Lake

Echo Park

Glendale Blvd

Clinton St

Laguna Ave

Crosby Pl

West Kensington Rd

Echo Park Ave

Belmont

finish

start

West Kensington Rd

Laveta Terrace

West Edgeware Rd

Douglas St

Carroll Ave

Bellevue Ave

Calumet Ave

101

Glendale Blvd

Temple St

Marion Ave

| 0 | 100 | 200 | 300 yards |
| 0 | 100 | 200 | 300 meters |

29 ECHO PARK AND ANGELINO HEIGHTS: AN UNEXPECTED SLICE OF VICTORIANA

BOUNDARIES: **Alvarado St., Sunset Blvd., Bellevue Ave.**
THOMAS GUIDE COORDINATES: **Map 634; D1**
DISTANCE: **Approx. 2 miles**
DIFFICULTY: **Moderate (includes stairways)**
PARKING: **Free street parking is available on Clinton St. (Pay attention to posted signs.)**

Echo Park is one of several East Side neighborhoods populated by that uniquely LA combination of Latino families and 20- to 30-something hipsters. Located immediately northwest of downtown, this hilly region features some gorgeous homes, many with excellent views, and is convenient to many of the modish shopping/dining destinations that have popped up in the area, particularly along Sunset and Silver Lake boulevards. Echo Park itself is also a draw—its picturesque lake is a convenient community gathering place and a distinctive focal point of the region. Perhaps the most fascinating feature of this neighborhood, the gorgeous Victorian homes of Angelino Heights, are located up on a hill just east of Echo Park Lake.

● Begin at the intersection of Clinton St. and Belmont Ave., where Clinton St. ends east of Alvarado St. Turn right to head south on Belmont. You'll pass a stairway at the end of Clinton, which leads down toward the Echo Park Lake.

● At the intersection of Bellevue Ave., turn left to follow the sidewalk that takes you to the steps leading down to Glendale Blvd. The walkway is marred somewhat by graffiti and litter, but it's nicely trimmed with bougainvillea and palm trees. Cross Glendale Blvd. at the bottom of the steps.

● Once across the street, follow the pathway on your left down into Echo Park and then bear right to continue on the path along the south end of the lake. Echo Park is a vibrant and scenic community center with a heavy Latino cultural influence; you may see a *paleta* (popsicle) salesman circling the lake with his cart. Mothers push strollers along the path, as kids take the paddle boats out for a ride and older gentlemen cast fishing lines out into the placid green water. At the far end of the lake, several jets of water spray high into the air. Continue to follow the path up the east side of the lake, parallel to Echo Park Ave.

● When you reach the paddle boat rental area about halfway up the east side of the lake, follow the stairs on your right out of the park and cross Echo Park Ave. at the crosswalk.

● Continue on Laguna Ave., heading northeast, and pass a church on your left. This is a modest residential street, populated mostly by older apartment buildings.

● Ascend the Crosby Pl. stairway on your right (opposite 867 Laguna Ave.). The concrete steps are heavily coated in graffiti and bordered by overgrowth, but this vantage point affords a great view of the lake behind you. At the top of the steps, continue straight on Crosby Pl. A striking gray Colonial Revival duplex sits on the southwest corner of Crosby Pl. and W. Kensington Rd. This is the first of many architecturally fascinating homes you will encounter as you continue on your walk through Angelino Heights.

● Turn left on W. Kensington Rd. Another charming Colonial Revival home sits at 1005 W. Kensington. In stark contrast, a deep orange, Spanish-style apartment building with a cactus garden in the front

Back Story: LA's Victorian Suburb

Before it was declared Los Angeles' very first Historic Preservation Overlay Zone in 1983, Angelino Heights had survived boom and bust. Developers William W. Stilson and Everett E. Hall created this residential subdivision in 1886 as one of the city's first suburbs—a unique housing tract composed of ornate Queen Anne and Eastlake Victorian homes that was conveniently located on the outskirts of LA's then-bustling downtown area. Unfortunately, a banking recession in 1888 put a stop to the development, leaving about 50 of these amazing homes to admire today; most of them are concentrated on Carroll and Kellam avenues. The 1300 block of Carroll Ave. is listed on the National Register of Historic Places for its heavy concentration of Victorians, most of which have been lovingly restored and maintained by the current owners.

Kensington Rd., which borders this timeless Victorian oasis, came to be populated with distinguished Craftsman houses during a second wave of development in the early 1900s. As a result, Angelino Heights now offers a rare selection of finely constructed, beautiful homes, and a combination of architectural styles that aren't found elsewhere in Los Angeles.

is right next door. Continue on W. Kensington Rd. as it curves to the right, crossing Laveta Terrace. The houses on this street become larger and more elaborate as you head farther uphill; many of the Craftsmans date back to the early 1900s. The first Victorian you encounter, at 892 W. Kensington Rd., looks incongruous among the many Craftsman and Colonial Revival homes.

● Turn right on Douglas St. and continue for about two blocks to W. Edgeware Rd. A somber Victorian, heavily shrouded by trees, on the southwest corner of Douglas and W. Edgeware, has the look of a haunted house.

● Turn left on W. Edgeware Rd. This street features a few historical Craftsman and Colonial Revival homes scattered among the mostly rundown apartment buildings that were built later in the 20th century. As the road curves to the south, a view of the nearby downtown skyscrapers opens up ahead.

● Turn right on Carroll Ave., where you'll be transported into another era. Developed as a suburban housing tract for Los Angeles' downtown professionals in the 1880s, the Queen Anne and Eastlake Victorian homes along the 1300 block of Carroll have been immaculately restored and maintained thanks to a devoted preservation effort, and they are now listed on the National Register of Historic Places. The juxtaposition of these intricately ornamented homes and the sleek downtown high-rises that lie immediately beyond is a sight to see. This street makes an excellent Halloween destination, as nearly all of the residents get into the spirit by decking out their old-fashioned homes with giant spider-webs and hanging dummies.

Victorian home in Angelino Heights

● At the end of Carroll Ave., turn left on W. Edgeware Rd., where the quality and main-tenance of the residences deteriorates rapidly. Head downhill toward the noisy 101 Freeway.

● Turn right on Bellevue Ave., which runs parallel to the freeway. As you cross Echo Park Ave., you'll see a swimming pool, part of the Echo Park Recreation Center, immediately adjacent to the freeway onramp. It seems like a bizarrely inappropriate location for a kids' pool. You also pass Echo Park Lake, on your right, and the rec center playground and picnic area, which are usually lively with some celebration or another, on your left.

● Cross Glendale Blvd. at the signal and then turn right on the other side to head toward the Clinton St. stairway you passed at the start of your walk. This is the sec-ond of three stairways along this block (the first was the Bellevue Ave. stairway you descended earlier).

● Ascend the Clinton St. steps, a double stairway that leads back to the junction of Clinton St. and Belmont Ave., where you began your journey.

route summary

1. Begin at the intersection of Clinton St. and Belmont Ave., and head south on Belmont Ave.
2. At the intersection of Bellevue Ave., turn left to follow the sidewalk that takes you to the steps leading down to Glendale Blvd.
3. Cross Glendale and follow the pathway on your left into Echo Park, and then bear right to continue on the path along the south and then east sides of the lake.
4. Exit the park at the stairs near the paddle boat rental area and cross Echo Park Blvd.
5. Walk northeast on Laguna Ave.
6. Ascend the Crosby Pl. stairway on your right (opposite 867 Laguna Ave.).
7. At the top of the steps, continue straight on Crosby Pl.
8. Turn left on W. Kensington Rd.
9. Turn right on Douglas St.
10. Turn left on W. Edgeware Rd.
11. Turn right on Carroll Ave.
12. Turn left on W. Edgeware Rd.
13. Turn right on Bellevue Ave.
14. Cross Glendale Blvd. at the signal and turn right on Glendale.
15. Ascend the Clinton St. stairway to return to your starting point.

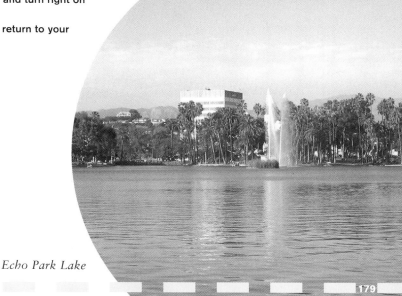

Echo Park Lake

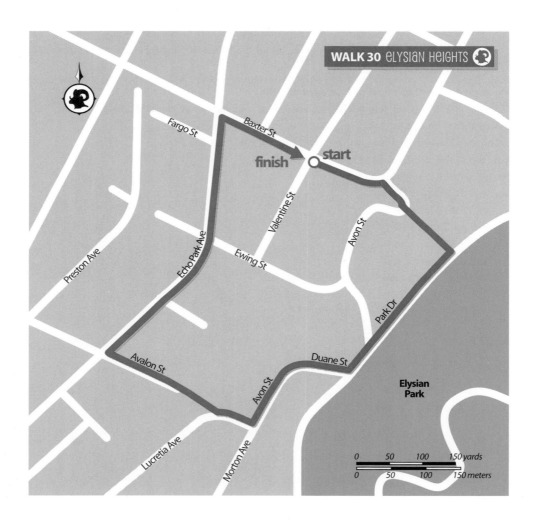

WALK 30 ELYSIAN HEIGHTS

Fargo St

Baxter St

finish   start

Valentine St

Avon St

Preston Ave

Echo Park Ave

Ewing St

Park Dr

Avalon St

Duane St

Elysian
Park

Avon St

Lucretia Ave

Morton Ave

0	50	100	150 yards
0	50	100	150 meters

30 ELYSIAN HEIGHTS: LOOKING DOWN ON LA'S OLDEST PUBLIC PARK

BOUNDARIES: **Alvarado St., Baxter St., Park Dr.**
THOMAS GUIDE COORDINATES: **Map 564; F6**
DISTANCE: **Approx. ¾ mile**
DIFFICULTY: **Moderate (includes stairways)**
PARKING: **Free street parking is available on Baxter St.**

Founded in 1781, Elysian Park is Los Angeles' second largest urban oasis (right behind Griffith Park). Its 600 acres are planted with native chaparral as well as eucalyptus and ficus trees. The park, which is home to Dodger Stadium, also features hiking trails, picnic areas, and playing fields for the nature-craving residents of central and eastern Los Angeles. The hilly neighborhood of Elysian Heights abuts the western border of the park, thus providing a delightful escape for residents who wish to forget for a little while that they live in one of the nation's most concrete-bound cities.

● Begin at the intersection of Valentine St. and Baxter St. (east of Echo Park Ave.) and head east toward the hill. An elementary school is on your right. This is a peaceful residential neighborhood; the cute, cottage-like homes on the left side of the street are lushly landscaped with assorted indigenous plant life: fruit trees, cactus, and more colorful floral varieties.

● Turn right on Avon St. Ascend the steps on your left, a very long, zigzagging stairway that appears to be carefully maintained—there are even street lights installed alongside the steps. On the hill above are a few modern homes. Pause every once in awhile to admire the stunning view behind you, which stretches from Century City to Griffith Park.

● Turn right at the top of the stairs onto Park Dr. Directly across the street is Elysian Park, a lush green basin with dirt paths winding down to the bottom. This 600-acre park features an arboretum, countless dirt hiking paths, and picnic areas. Through the eucalyptus trees to the southeast, you can catch an excellent view of downtown.

Joggers and dog-walkers travel the dirt path just a few yards below, and if you're so inclined, you can hop down the short slope and join them in exploring this big, rustic oasis.

● Continue along Park Dr. to Duane St. and turn right. Duane has the feel of a narrow country lane as it curves downhill to the left and turns into Avon St.

● Turn right on Lucretia Ave., and just after the road curves to the left, look for a narrow sidewalk on your right; follow it to the next stairway, nearly as long as the one you ascended earlier, which zigzags down to Avalon St. As you descend, admire more fabulous views all the way to the coast (on a clear day) to the west, and to the San Gabriel Mountains to the northeast.

● Continue straight on Avalon St. for one block to Echo Park Ave.

● Turn right on Echo Park Ave. The next few blocks are considerably less idyllic than the elevated portion of this walk; some of the houses are rundown, and the commercial options don't extend much beyond a liquor store and a hair salon.

● When you reach the elementary school near your starting point, turn right on Baxter St., and follow it back to the intersection with Valentine St., where you began.

route summary

1. Begin at the intersection of Valentine St. and Baxter St., (east of Echo Park Ave.) and head east.

2. Turn right on Avon St. and ascend the long, zigzagging staircase on your left.

3. Turn right at the top of the stairs onto Park Dr.

4. Turn right on Duane St. and follow it as it curves to the left and turns into Avon St.

5. Turn right on Lucretia Ave., and just after the road curves to the left, look for a narrow sidewalk on your right—follow it to the next stairway and descend.

6. Continue straight on Avalon St. for one block to Echo Park Ave.

7. Turn right on Echo Park Ave.

8. Turn right on Baxter St., and follow it back to the intersection with Valentine St.

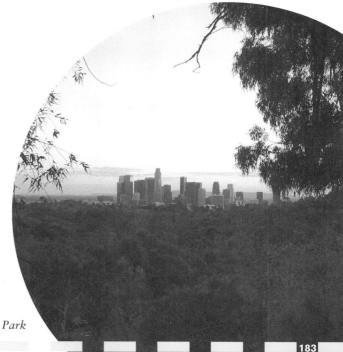

View of downtown LA through Elysian Park

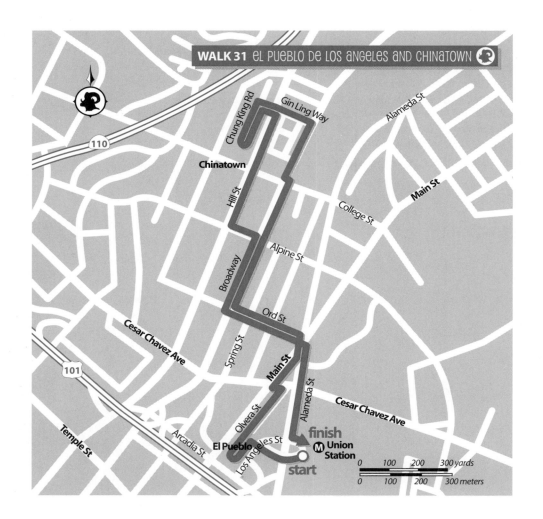

WALK 31 EL PUEBLO DE LOS ANGELES AND CHINATOWN

Chung King Rd

Gin Ling Way

Alameda St

110

Chinatown

Hill St

College St

Main St

Broadway

Alpine St

Ord St

Cesar Chavez Ave

101

Spring St

Main St

Alameda St

Cesar Chavez Ave

Temple St

Olvera St

Arcadia St

El Pueblo

Los Angeles St

finish
M Union
Station

start

0   100   200   300 yards

0   100   200   300 meters

31 EL PUEBLO DE LOS ANGELES AND CHINATOWN: WHERE HISTORY, CULTURE, AND TOURISM COLLIDE

BOUNDARIES: **101 Freeway, Alameda St., 110 Freeway**
THOMAS GUIDE COORDINATES: **Map 634: G3**
DISTANCE: **Approx. 2 miles**
DIFFICULTY: **Easy**
PARKING: **There are paid parking lots on Alameda St. and Los Angeles St. There is also limited metered parking on Alameda, across from Union Station, as well as on surrounding side streets, but it's easiest to take the Metro public rail system to this walk. After all, it does begin at the hub of LA's (admittedly limited) subway system.**
NEAREST METRO STATION: **Union Station, 800 N. Alameda St.**

This walk is about as diverse as it gets, exploring both El Pueblo de Los Angeles, home to the area's first Mexican settlers, and Chinatown, which is a thriving hub for the city's Chinese-American community and a standard tourist attraction. Both neighborhoods now serve as enduring tributes to the history of the settlers and immigrants who have contributed to the development of the greater Los Angeles multicultural society. Your journey begins at one of the city's most recognizable Art Deco landmarks and its central hub for public transit, Union Station.

● Begin at Union Station at 800 N. Alameda St. This wonderfully romantic building was established in 1939 and combines the influence of Art Deco and Spanish Colonial Revival architecture to splendid effect. If you traveled here by car, walk through the colossal arched entryway and spend a few minutes taking in the gorgeous painted ceilings, intricate inlaid marble floors and walls, ornate black iron chandeliers, and historic Art Deco furnishings of America's "last great rail station." On the north side of the station is an enclosed patio with a colorful tiled wall fountain. Union Station's resident upscale eatery, Traxx restaurant and bar, offers al fresco dining on this patio.

● After you've finished exploring the station, exit through the south doorway and walk across the brick-paved plaza to the Metropolitan Water District Building to admire the lovely circular fountain out front, which is tiled in a brilliant fish-scale design. Return to the plaza and head west toward Alameda St.

- Follow Los Angeles St. across Alameda to enter El Pueblo de Los Angeles, the approximate site of the original town founded by settlers in 1781, back when California still belonged to Mexico. You'll pass the grassy area known as Father Serra Park, which features a statue of the beloved Franciscan priest.

- Continue straight along the pedestrian walkway Paseo de la Plaza. As you approach the gathering center of the plaza—an enormous gazebo that acts as a stage for mariachi bands and street performers—you pass the Biscailuz Building on your right. This former home of the Mexican Consulate General now houses the Mexican Cultural Institute. A vibrant mural by Leo Politi, *Blessing of the Animals*, graces one wall of the building.

- Head south across the plaza to check out some of El Pueblo's historic buildings. At the corner of Main St. and Arcadia St. are the Masonic Hall (established in 1858); Los Angeles' first theatrical house, the Merced Theatre (established 1870); and the Pico House, an extravagant, Italianate luxury hotel commissioned by the last governor of Mexican California, Pío Pico, in 1870. Los Angeles' first fire station, Firehouse No.1 (established in 1884), sits at the southeast corner of the plaza; the restored building is now a museum for late 19th century firefighting memorabilia (free tours are available).

- Walk northeast back across the plaza and look for the entrance to Olvera St., which is identified by a large brown cross. The rich aroma of leather emanates from the purse and belt vendor stalls that crowd the entrance. This one-block pedestrian alley is a popular tourist attraction designed to re-create the type of thriving marketplace you might find in Tijuana or Ensenada. At 10 Olvera St., you come to the Avila Adobe, the oldest existing house in Los Angeles, built by Don Francisco Avila in 1818 (free tours are available). As you continue through the alley, you pass an eclectic mix of stalls and shops selling souvenirs, western clothing, jewelry, Mexican artwork, candies, *pan dulce*, and other treats. If you prefer to skip the snack food stalls and sit down for a full, authentic Mexican meal, Casa la Golondrina, at 17 Olvera St., is a popular spot.

- You emerge from Olvera St. onto Cesar E. Chavez Ave. Turn left here.

- In less than a block, turn right on Main St. and follow it to where Main merges with Alameda St.

- Turn left on Alameda, and then immediately turn left again onto Ord St. Philippe the Original occupies the northwest corner of this intersection. Even if you don't plan to eat at the legendary deli and French dip slinger, you ought to step inside to check out the joint's singular ambience. The interior appears to have changed little since it was established in 1908; sawdust covers the floors and long, communal picnic tables lined with benches occupy most of the space. The building is huge, offering private booth seating in the rear of the first floor and several private rooms upstairs. In addition to the legendary sandwich, you can purchase all manner of deli items behind the busy counter, as well as Philippe's famous 9¢ cup of coffee. Public restrooms are also available here.

- Exit back onto Ord. St. and turn right to continue west for three short blocks to Broadway.

- Turn right on Broadway, staying on the east side of the street; you're now on Chinatown's main drag. As you head north on Broadway, you pass jewelry and clothing stores, a pungent fish market, and several tiny shops selling Chinese dried goods and spices.

- Cross Alpine St. and arrive at the 800 block of Broadway, which is home to several malls—Dynasty Center, Chinatown Plaza, and Saigon Plaza. The plaza most worth poking your head into is Saigon, an outdoor collection of vendor stalls

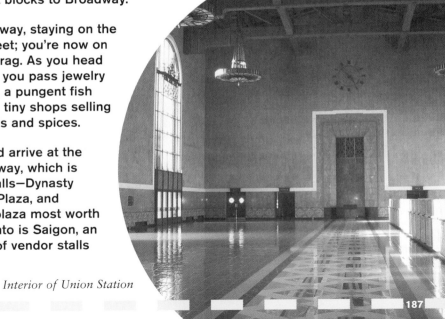

Interior of Union Station

selling clothing, shoes, slippers, and a delectable array of deep-fried treats.

- When you reach College St., cross to the west side of Broadway and continue north. You pass a beautiful, tiled mural next door to the Big China Restaurant, at 911 Broadway.

- Pass the first gateway you come to, which leads into an alley, and continue to the East Gate, the magnificent entryway to Chinatown's Central Plaza. The colorful wooden portal is an example of Neo-Chinese architecture, which is carried through in the gorgeous tile work and gaily painted balconies inside the plaza.

- Turn left to enter through the East Gate, following Gin Ling Way into the Central Plaza. The Wonder Food Bakery is just inside the entrance on your left, and a lovely fountain trickles on your right. Gin Ling Way is hung with red and white paper lanterns and lined with tourist shops selling a variety of Chinese tchotchkes. Gin Ling Way is also home to Mountain Bar, whose dimly lit, deep red interior attracts artists and hipsters. On your left, just before Mei Ling Way, you pass a massive wishing well sculpture that dates back to 1939; toss your coins toward little signs representing "Health," "Money," "Love," and other good fortunes.

BACK STORY: EL PUEBLO AND CHINATOWN

Interestingly enough, both El Pueblo de Los Angeles and Chinatown have been moved from their original sites. The actual location where Mexican settlers established their village in 1781 was closer to the Los Angeles River, just east of where Union Station stands today, but flooding in 1818 forced them to move to higher ground—the current site of El Pueblo. For its part, the original neighborhood known as Chinatown was rudely displaced to make way for construction of Union Station in the 1930s. The Chinese immigrants eventually developed the thriving community a few blocks to the northwest in what is now more appropriately referred to as "New Chinatown."

As you cross Mei Ling Way, look to your left to see the five-tier pagoda atop Hop Louie restaurant and bar. This distinctive Chinatown landmark was constructed in 1941.

● Cross Hill St. and continue into Chinatown's West Plaza by way of Chung King Ct. Chung King Ct. dead-ends at Chung King Rd., another pedestrian walkway that has attracted a spate of artists in recent years, making the West Plaza a destination for hot new gallery openings.

● Turn left on Chung King Rd. to explore some of the galleries before returning to Chung King Ct.

● Exit West Plaza by way of Chung King Ct. and turn right on Hill St. to head south. If you've managed to hold out this long, Foo Chow, a restaurant on the southwest corner of Chung King Ct. and Hill St., is an excellent place to stop for a generous helping of noodles, seafood, or moo-shu for not a lot of money. On the east side of Hill St., just south of Gin Ling Way, there is an empty lot in which large white letters have been erected to spell "Chinatownland"—a cheeky tribute to the original Hollywoodland sign above Beachwood Canyon.

● Cross College St. and continue south on Hill St., admiring the view of the downtown skyline straight ahead. At 825 Hill St. is the Chinese United Methodist Church; appropriately enough, this house of worship incorporates elements of both Chinese- and Western-style architecture.

Hop Louie restaurant and bar

189

- Turn left on Alpine St. and continue for one block back to Broadway.

- Turn right on Broadway, but this time remain on the west side of the street. Cathay Bank, the first Chinese-American-owned bank in Southern California, sits on the southwest corner of Alpine and Broadway. Continue south on Broadway, passing the Far East Plaza on your right. This shopping mall is home to numerous restaurants serving a variety of Far East regional cuisines, as well as to the Wing Hop Fung Ginseng and China Products Center, which sells an abundance of herbs, teas, and Chinese arts and crafts.

- Turn left on Ord St., retracing your steps for a few blocks back to Alameda St.

- Turn right on Alameda. On the east side of the street, at 900 N. Alameda, look for the imposing Mission/Spanish Revival façade of the U.S. Post Office Terminal Annex, which was designed by Gilbert S. Underwood in 1938.

- Cross Cesar E. Chavez Ave. to return to your starting point at Union Station.

POINTS OF INTEREST

Traxx 800 N. Alameda St. (inside Union Station), Los Angeles, CA 90012, 213-625-1999

Firehouse No. 1 134 Paseo de la Plaza, Los Angeles, CA 90012, 213-628-1274

Avila Adobe 10 Olvera St., Los Angeles, CA 90012, 213-628-1274

Casa la Golondrina 17 Olvera St., Los Angeles, CA 90012, 213-628-4349

Philippe the Original 1001 N. Alameda St., Los Angeles, CA 90012, 213-628-3781

Mountain Bar 475 Gin Ling Way, Los Angeles, CA 90012, 213-625-7500

Hop Louie 950 Mei Ling Way (inside Central Plaza), Los Angeles, CA 90012, 213-628-4244

Wing Hop Fung Ginseng and China Products Center 727 N. Broadway, Los Angeles, CA 90012, 213-626-7200

Foo Chow 949 N. Hill St., Los Angeles, CA 90012, 213-485-1294

route summary

1. Begin at Union Station, at 800 N. Alameda St., exit the station through the south doorway, and head west through the plaza toward Alameda St.

2. Follow Los Angeles St. across Alameda to enter El Pueblo de Los Angeles.

3. Continue straight along the pedestrian walkway known as Paseo de la Plaza.

4. Head southwest across the plaza to check out some of El Pueblo's historic buildings.

5. Walk northeast back across the plaza and continue through Olvera St.

6. Emerge from Olvera St. onto Cesar E. Chavez Ave. and turn left.

7. Turn right on Main St. and follow it to where it merges with Alameda St.

8. Turn left on Alameda St.

9. Turn left on Ord St.

10. Turn right on Broadway, staying on the east side of the street.

11. At College St., cross to the west side of Broadway and continue north.

12. Turn left to enter Central Plaza through the East Gate, following Gin Ling Way.

13. Cross Hill St. and continue into Chinatown's West Plaza by way of Chung King Ct. Chung King Ct. dead-ends at Chung King Rd.

14. Turn left on Chung King Rd. to explore some of the galleries before retracing your steps to Chung King Ct.

15. Follow Chung King Ct. back to exit the West Plaza and turn right on Hill St. to head south.

16. Turn left on Alpine St.

17. Turn right on Broadway, remaining on the west side of the street.

18. Turn left on Ord St., retracing your steps for a few blocks back to Alameda St.

19. Turn right on Alameda.

20. Cross Cesar E. Chavez Ave. to return to your starting point at Union Station.

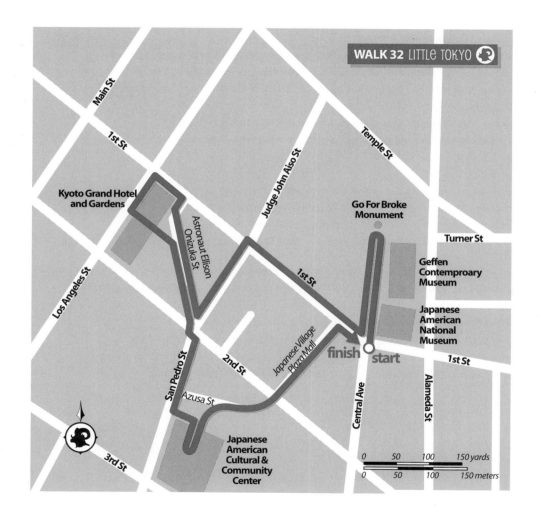

WALK 32 LITTLE TOKYO

Main St

1st St

Temple St

Kyoto Grand Hotel
and Gardens

Go For Broke
Monument

Turner St

Judge John Aiso St

Astronaut Ellison
Onizuka St

Geffen
Contemproary
Museum

1st St

Japanese
American
National
Museum

San Pedro St

2nd St

Japanese Village
Plaza Mall

finish   start

1st St

Azusa St

Central Ave

Alameda St

Japanese
American
Cultural &
Community
Center

Los Angeles St

3rd St

0   50   100   150 yards
0   50   100   150 meters

32 LITTLE TOKYO: A PROUD TRIBUTE TO JAPANESE IMMIGRANT HISTORY

BOUNDARIES: **Temple St., Los Angeles St., 3rd St., Alameda St.**
THOMAS GUIDE COORDINATES: **Map 634; G4**
DISTANCE: **Approx. ¾ mile**
DIFFICULTY: **Easy**
PARKING: **Metered street parking is available on 1st St.**
NEAREST METRO STATION: **Civic Center, 1st St. and Hill St. (Red Line)**

Located in downtown Los Angeles, just south of the 101 Freeway and next door to the artists loft district, is Little Tokyo, a neighborhood that simultaneously projects multicultural urban cool while retaining its ties to Japanese-American history. There's plenty to draw locals and tourists alike to this region, such as authentic Japanese eateries too numerous to count, spas offering affordable shiatsu treatments, shops selling colorful knickknacks, the Japanese American National Museum, and even the Geffen Contemporary extension of the Museum of Contemporary Art.

● Begin at the intersection of Central Ave. and 1st. St., where Central Ave. ends and transforms into an open pedestrian plaza. On the east side of the clearing is the site of the Japanese American National Museum, a graceful sandstone, metal, and glass building that was designed by Gyo Obata, who also designed the Air and Space Museum in Washington, D.C. Just across the plaza, the National Center for the Preservation of Democracy is housed in a lovely old brick building that was established in 1925 and originally was the site of the Nishi Hongwanzi Buddhist Temple.

● Head north through the plaza toward the Geffen Contemporary branch of the Museum of Contemporary Art (MOCA), the site for installation pieces that are too large to fit in the museum's California Plaza location downtown. After you pass the warehouse-like home of MOCA's easternmost satellite, you'll come to the Go For Broke monument, which commemorates more than 16,000 Japanese-American veterans of World War II who voluntarily went to Europe and the Pacific Rim to fight for the same country that sent their families to internment camps back in the States.

Surviving veterans volunteer as guides at the monument, and if you have the time to talk to one of these incredibly brave and patriotic men, you'll no doubt be amazed at the stories he has to tell.

● Return to the intersection of Central and 1st and turn right to head west for one block on 1st St., passing a crowded collection of Japanese sweet shops, sushi restaurants, and shiatsu spas. Glance downward along the north side to see Little Tokyo's history engraved in the pavement—this is Little Tokyo's Historic District.

● Turn left on San Pedro St. (it's called Judge John Aiso St. in the opposite direction). As you continue south, you'll come to the site of Seiji Kunishima's *Stonerise* sculpture, a massive art piece composed of roughly textured black granite blocks, which sits in a quiet garden on the north side of the Union Bank building.

● At the northwest corner of San Pedro and 2nd St. is the entrance to Weller Ct., also known as Astronaut Ellison S. Onizuka St., for the first Japanese-American astronaut. This pedestrian street is marked by Shinkichi Tajiri's *Friendship Knot* sculpture. As you walk through the court, you'll pass Marukai Market, a large grocery store where you can purchase all manner of authentic Japanese goodies. About halfway through the court is a replica of the *Challenger* space shuttle, aboard which Onizuka launched his final space mission.

● At the end of Weller Ct./Onizuka St., turn left on Los Angeles St. and proceed to the main entrance of the Kyoto Grand Hotel and Gardens. Enter the lobby and take the elevator on your right up to the garden level. You'll emerge into a lovely rooftop Japanese garden; the two-level oasis features waterfalls and walking paths, and provides an excellent view of the downtown skyline to the southwest.

● Return to the elevator booth, but instead of re-boarding, follow the sign for Weller Ct., descending the stairs on the east side of the garden. You'll walk down through a multilevel food court offering udon, curry, and other Japanese fare. Return to ground level in Weller Ct. and turn right to head back to the intersection of San Pedro St. and 2nd St.

- Cross 2nd and then cross to the east side of San Pedro St. and turn right to head south. In front of the bank on the southeast corner is a bronze statue of prominent Japanese farmer Sontoku (Kinjiro) Ninomiya, sometimes known as the "peasant sage of Japan."

- After crossing the Azusa St. alley, you come to the Japanese American Cultural and Community Center. Enter the spacious, brick-paved plaza, designed by Isamu Noguchi. The imposing concrete façade of the center lies directly to the south.

- Enter the center through the massive glass doors and take the elevator down to the basement level, where you can explore the beautiful James Irvine Japanese Garden, a carefully tended paradise that lies in stark contrast to the imposing concrete building that towers above.

- Return to ground level and walk back across the plaza to the Azusa St. alley. Follow the short alley through to 2nd St.

- Cross 2nd. St. and continue through the Japanese Village Plaza Mall, bearing right at the split to continue on the path toward 1st St. This is the heart of Little Tokyo's shopping district, offering sushi and noodle cafes, shabu shabu dining, knickknack shops, shiatsu massage, sweets, and plenty of other opportunities to indulge yourself.

- After grabbing a snack, meal, or massage in the plaza, exit onto 1st St., where you'll find yourself back at your starting point at the intersection of Central Ave.

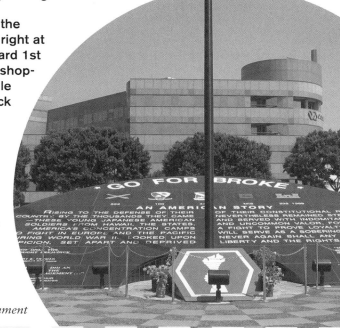

Go For Broke monument

WALKING L.A.

POINTS OF Interest

Japanese American National Museum 369 E. 1st St., Los Angeles, CA 90012, 213-625-0414

Geffen Contemporary 152 N. Central Ave., Los Angeles, CA 90013, 213-626-6222

Kypto Grand Hotel and Gardens 120 S. Los Angeles St., Los Angeles, CA 90012, 213-629-1200

Japanese American Cultural and Community Center 244 S. San Pedro St., Ste 505, Los Angeles, CA 90012, 213-628-2725

196

route summary

1. Begin at the intersection of Central Ave. and 1st St. and head north through the plaza to the Go For Broke monument.

2. Return to the intersection of Central Ave. and 1st St. and turn right on 1st St.

3. Turn left on San Pedro St.

4. Enter Weller Ct. (a.k.a. Astronaut Ellison S. Onizuka St.) at the northwest corner of San Pedro and 2nd St.

5. At the end of Weller Ct., turn left on Los Angeles St. Enter the lobby of the Kyoto Grand Hotel and Gardens and take the elevator on your right up to the garden level.

6. From the rooftop garden, follow the sign for Weller Ct., descending the stairs on the east side of the garden. Turn right at the bottom to head back to the intersection of San Pedro St. and 2nd St.

7. Cross 2nd and then cross to the east side of San Pedro St. and turn right to head south.

8. After crossing the Azusa St. alley, enter the plaza of the Japanese American Culture and Community Center.

9. Enter the center and take the elevator down to the James Irvine Japanese Garden at basement level.

10. Return to ground level and walk back across the plaza to the Azusa St. alley. Follow the short alley to 2nd St.

11. Cross 2nd St. and continue through the Japanese Village Plaza Mall, bearing right at the split to continue on the path toward 1st St.

12. Exit the mall onto 1st St., returning to your starting point at the intersection of Central Ave.

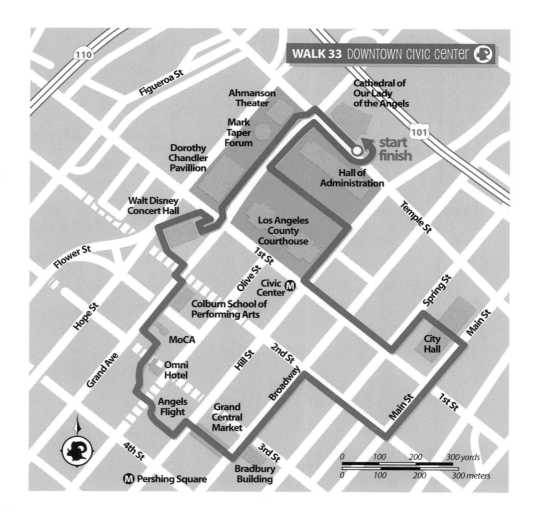

110

Figueroa St

Ahmanson
Theater

Cathedral of
Our Lady
of the Angels

Mark
Taper
Forum

101

Dorothy
Chandler
Pavillion

start
finish

Hall of
Administration

Walt Disney
Concert Hall

Temple St

Los Angeles
County
Courthouse

Flower St

1st St

Olive St

Civic
Center M

Spring St

Hope St

Colburn School of
Performing Arts

Main St

MoCA

City
Hall

Grand Ave

Omni
Hotel

Hill St

2nd St

Angels
Flight

Grand
Central
Market

Broadway

Main St

1st St

4th St

3rd St

0   100   200   300 yards
0   100   200   300 meters

M Pershing Square

Bradbury
Building

33 DOWNTOWN CIVIC CENTER: REVITALIZATION IN THE WORKS

BOUNDARIES: 101 Freeway, Hope St., Main St., 4th St.
THOMAS GUIDE COORDINATES: Map 634; F3
DISTANCE: Approx. 2 miles
DIFFICULTY: Moderate (includes stairways)
PARKING: Like every building downtown, the Cathedral of Our Lady of Angels, where this route begins, requires that you pay for parking. Your best bet is to do this walk on a weekend or on a weekday after 4 P.M., when you can park for a fairly reasonable flat fee. Provided that you attend Sunday Mass, you can park for three hours for free. Alternatively, you can take the Metro Red Line to the Civic Center stop, and then walk a block north to your starting point at the cathedral. Alternatively, you can always try your luck with metered parking on the surrounding streets.
NEAREST METRO STATION: Civic Center, 1st St. and Hill St. (Red Line)

The Civic Center, as the area of downtown just south of the 101 Freeway and just east of the 110 is called, has been subject to some eccentric developments over the past few years as part of a revitalization effort, and the overhaul is far from over. Over the next several years, numerous ugly parking structures will be leveled to make way for more commercial, residential, retail, and hotel space. Presently, the effect of all this expansion is occasionally successful—as in the case of the majestic Walt Disney Concert Hall. At other times, it's discordant—witness the decidedly ungraceful design of the Cathedral of Our Lady of Angels. This walk explores these new additions to the downtown cityscape, as well as the institutions that form the city's historic core, such as City Hall and Grand Central Market.

● Begin at the Cathedral of Our Lady of Angels, at 555 W. Temple St. Regardless of whether you park in the structure or walk from the Metro station, enter the cathedral grounds via the lower courtyard, which is graced with a waterfall fountain. Ascend the stairs into the main courtyard to access the cathedral itself, as well as a little cafe and gift shop. Before proceeding toward the church, wander to the northeast corner of the upper courtyard, where you'll discover an interesting sculpture garden featuring an assortment of wild and domestic creatures. The cathedral looms formidably ahead. Architect Rafael Moneo constructed the massive edifice out of adobe-colored concrete, creating an oddly striated effect with his layered formation of the outer walls.

Enter the cathedral by way of the great bronze doors on the left side of the façade. The starkly modern interior feels refreshingly cool on hot days and carries through the exterior theme of neutral tones in stone, wood, and marble. Filtered sunlight enters through the gray-tinted Spanish alabaster windows. Take a few moments to explore, sticking to the perimeter of the building if there is a service underway, and you'll find a collection of sculptures and framed oil paintings that are dwarfed by the dimensions of the interior space. The most striking pieces of art are the hand-painted tapestries lining the walls of the inner sanctuary; they portray a sampling of the Catholic community—young and old people of various ethnicities. (The cathedral offers free group tours.)

- After exploring the cathedral, exit back into the plaza the same way you came in, return to street level, and turn right to head west along Temple St.

- Cross Grand Ave., and then cross to the south side of Temple so that you are on the southwest corner of the intersection. Ascend the stairs to reach the collection of the-aters that comprise the Music Center complex.

- Turn left at the top of the stairs to walk through the Los Angeles Times Garden Courtyard, which is not so much a garden as a paved walkway between towering concrete columns. On your right is the Ahmanson Theatre and then the Mark Taper Forum, a striking cylindrical theater decorated with an abstract bas-relief. Note that there are public restrooms on your left.

After passing the reflecting pools that front the Mark Taper, you emerge into the main courtyard of the Music Center. The classy outdoor Pinot Grill operates in the evenings here, and you can also grab a quick, inexpensive bite at the Spotlight Cafe. The centerpiece of the plaza is an elevated dancing fountain built around an expressive and semi-religious sculpture entitled *Peace on Earth*. This large monument was dedicated by artist Jacques Lipchitz in 1969 as "a symbol of peace to the peoples of the world," according to the inscription on the base of the fountain. Take a few minutes to enjoy your vantage point in the midst of the Music Center complex. To the west, you can see the glass and steel Department of Water and Power building, flanked by its own magnificent high-spouting fountains. The distinctive City Hall tower (established in 1929), which incorporates classical and Art Deco design elements to elegant effect, rises beyond the sunken parkway directly to the southeast.

Before descending the stairway to Grand Ave. on the east side of the fountain, take a second to admire the metal sculpture of an open doorway by Robert Graham. The piece is called *Dance Door* and features a bas-relief of nude dancers reminiscent of Degas' ballerinas.

- At the bottom of the stairs, turn right on Grand. Pass the county courthouse on your left just before reaching 1st St., at which point the burnished, mellifluous wings of Frank Gehry's Walt Disney Concert Hall come into view. This world-renowned architectural masterpiece is now the permanent home of the Los Angeles Philharmonic. (For information about tours of Disney Hall, call 213-972-4399.)

- Cross 1st St. and enter the lobby through the glass doors on the east side of the building (facing Grand Ave.). The lobby is a study in curved surfaces—white-painted walls and ceilings with blond wood finishing. This is a tourist spot, so you'll find another gift shop and cafe here. Self-guided audio tours of the architectural highlights of the concert hall are available for a small fee.

- Exit Disney Hall back onto Grand Ave. and then turn left to backtrack slightly to the corner of 1st St. Turn left on 1st St., remaining on the same side of the street as the concert hall.

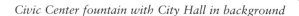

Civic Center fountain with City Hall in background

- Continue west on 1st for almost one block. Just before reaching Hope St., turn left to follow the stairway up to the community park hidden behind the concert hall. This garden is lovely and green, with plentiful shade trees and chairs to rest on. Continue to walk through the park to its centerpiece, a gently burbling fountain in the shape of a giant rose. This unique sculpture is covered in a mosaic of broken blue-and-white china pieces, and was designed by Gehry as a tribute to Lillian Disney on behalf of her children and grandchildren.

- Proceed toward the far end of the park and then turn left to cut through the charming outdoor Children's Amphitheatre. Descend the stairway back down to Grand Ave. and turn right.

- Cross 2nd St. and then cross Grand Ave. so that you are on the same side of the street as the Colburn School of Performing Arts. Continue south on Grand to reach the brick-colored walls of the Museum of Contemporary Art (MOCA). The museum's roofline is eccentrically punctuated with pyramid-shaped skylights.

- Turn left to enter MOCA's outdoor plaza, which is identified by a looming sculpture that is essentially a top-heavy junk pile of wrecked airplane parts.

- Turn right to follow the narrow courtyard built around a long strip of reflecting pool and shaded by magnolia trees, passing the Omni Hotel on your left. As the plaza opens up, you'll find yourself overlooking the spectacular Watercourt fountain, which doubles as a stage for free outdoor concerts during the summer. (Visit www.grand-performances.org for more information.)

- Descend either the escalator or the stairway to your right, which deposits you in a covered hallway of numerous lunch-hour spots for the suit-and-tie crowd. You can grab a bite here, but you'd be better off choosing something more interesting from the variety at the Grand Central Market, which you will come to shortly. Turn right to emerge into the light on the same level of the Watercourt fountain.

- Walk around the front of the Watercourt, and then look for the stairway on your right that leads to the park below. Descend the first set of steps, and then continue down the next long stairway, which runs parallel to the sometimes operational Angels

Flight funicular. The sloping grassy park on your right is often populated with some of the city's homeless.

- At the bottom of the stairs, cross Hill St. to reach the entrance of Grand Central Market, LA's famous open-air market (open seven days a week), founded in 1917 and still offering a rich variety of culinary delights, including pizza, Thai, Chinese, burgers, sandwiches, ice cream, fresh-squeezed juices, Salvadorian, or any number of Mexican dining options. You can easily grab a sustaining meal for less than five bucks. Walk all the way through the market until you emerge onto Broadway.

- Turn left on Broadway. At the southeast corner of Broadway and 3rd St. is the Bradbury Building, which was designed by George H. Wyman in the 1890s. You must check out the inside of this architectural landmark, which is open to the public. The interior is illuminated by natural light filtering through the translucent domed roof high above the atrium. The elaborate stairways are composed of cast iron in an eclectic Victorian design. You may recognize the distinctive surroundings from the climactic fight scene in *Blade Runner*.

- Return to the street and continue northeast along Broadway. This part of town is rather shabby compared to the business district surrounding the Music Center, but it offers its share of interesting sites. For example, you'll notice the delightfully tacky Guadalupe Wedding Chapel, featuring a Romanesque façade ornamented with faux Corinthian columns—very Vegas—on the west side of the street just after you cross 3rd St. As you approach 2nd St., check out the Los Angeles Times parking structure on your

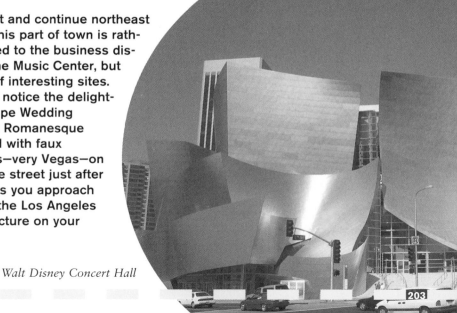

Walt Disney Concert Hall

203

right, which features an elaborate bas-relief artwork depicting a stylized history of California's colonization.

● Turn right on 2nd St. The new home of the LAPD headquarters (which may be under construction when you visit) is on your left. Pit Fire Pizza Company, a very good bet for a lunch of fresh salads and mouthwatering pizza and panini, is located on the southeast corner of 2nd and Main St. Across from Pit Fire, at 114 E. 2nd St., is St. Vibiana's Cathedral (dedicated in 1876). The cathedral has been damaged by an earthquake and threatened with demolition in the last century, but it still stands today as the result of passionate preservation efforts.

● Turn left on Main St. The Caltrans headquarters is on your right. The extraordinary (and imposing) glass and steel building occupies an entire block and was designed by prestigious architect Thom Mayne. An enormous 1-0-0 looms above the street, marking the building's address on Main St.

● Cross 1st St. and proceed to the public entrance to City Hall, on your left. The attractive Art Deco building is distinguished by its white tower; the concrete used for its construction is said to have been made from sand taken from each of California's 58 counties. Enter the building, get a visitor's badge from security, and take the elevator to the third floor, where you can admire the gorgeous, inlaid marble floor and the tile ceilings of the rotunda. Next, take the elevator up to the observation deck on the 27th floor, where you can admire 360-degree views of the city.

● After taking in the vista, return to ground level and exit the west-facing doors onto Spring St. Turn left on Spring.

● Turn right on 1st St., passing the Los Angeles Times building on your left, and then the Los Angeles County Law Library on your right as you make your way uphill.

● After crossing Hill St., turn right to head northeast on Hill.

● Pass the entrance to the county courthouse, and then turn left into the pleasant public park that runs between the courthouse and the Hall of Administration. Continue northwest through the park. At the far end, there is a magnificent circular fountain that projects a refreshing mist over the surrounding benches—a lovely place to take one last break before the end of the walk.

- On the other side of the fountain, ascend the stairs back up to Grand Ave. and turn right.

- Continue for a half block to Temple St. and turn right to return to your starting point at the cathedral.

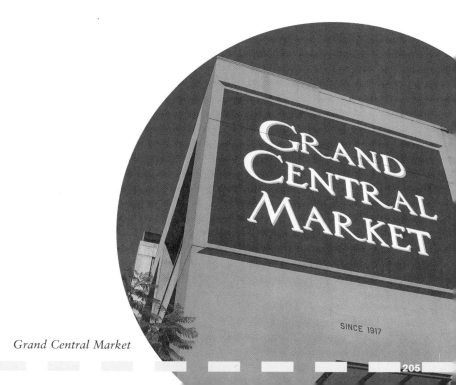

Grand Central Market

POINTS OF Interest

Cathedral of Our Lady of Angels 555 W. Temple St., Los Angeles, CA 90012,
213-680-5200

Music Center (Dorothy Chandler Pavilion, Ahmanson Theatre, Mark Taper Forum)
135 N. Grand Ave., Los Angeles, CA 90012, 213-972-7211

Walt Disney Concert Hall 111 S. Grand Ave., Los Angeles, CA 90012, 213-972-7211

Museum of Contemporary Art 250 S. Grand Ave., Los Angeles, CA 90012, 213-626-6222

Omni Hotel 251 S. Olive St., Los Angeles, CA 90012, 213-671-3300

Grand Central Market 317 S. Broadway St., Los Angeles, CA 90012, 213-624-2378

Pit Fire Pizza Company 108 W. 2nd St., Los Angeles, CA 90012, 213-808-1200

City Hall 200 N. Spring St. Los Angeles, CA 90012, 213-473-7001

route summary

1. Begin at the Cathedral of Our Lady of Angels on Temple St. between Grand Ave. and Hill St.
2. Explore the cathedral and then exit the courtyard and turn right on Temple St.
3. Cross Grand Ave., cross to the south side of Temple, and then ascend the stairs to the Music Center complex.
4. Turn left and cross through the Music Center plaza.
5. Descend the stairs on the east side of plaza back down to Grand Ave.
6. Turn right on Grand.
7. Cross 1st St. and enter the Walt Disney Hall lobby through the doors on Grand Ave.
8. Exit back onto Grand and turn left to return to the corner of 1st St., and then turn left on 1st.
9. Ascend the stairway on your left just before Hope St. and walk through the elevated park.
10. At far end of park, turn left to cut through the Children's Amphitheatre, and then descend the stairs back down to Grand Ave.
11. Cross 2nd St., cross Grand Ave., and then continue south on Grand.
12. Turn left to enter the MOCA outdoor plaza.
13. Turn right to walk through a narrow courtyard, emerging into the main plaza above the Watercourt fountain.
14. Descend the escalator on your right and turn right at the bottom.
15. Walk around the front of the Watercourt fountain and descend the stairs on the east side of the plaza.
16. At the bottom of the stairs, cross Hill St. and then walk through Grand Central Market.
17. Turn left on Broadway St. and then enter the Bradbury Building on the southeast corner of Broadway and 3rd St.
18. Return to Broadway and continue north.
19. Turn right on 2nd St.
20. Turn left on Main St.
21. Cross 1st St. and enter City Hall on your left. Visit the rotunda on the third floor and the observation deck on the 27th floor, then return to street level and exit the building's west-facing doors onto Spring St. Turn left on Spring.
22. Turn right on 1st St.
23. Turn right on Hill St.
24. Turn left to cut through the park between the county courthouse and the Hall of Administration.
24. Ascend the stairs back up to Grand Ave. and turn right.
25. Turn right on Temple St. to return to your starting point at the cathedral.

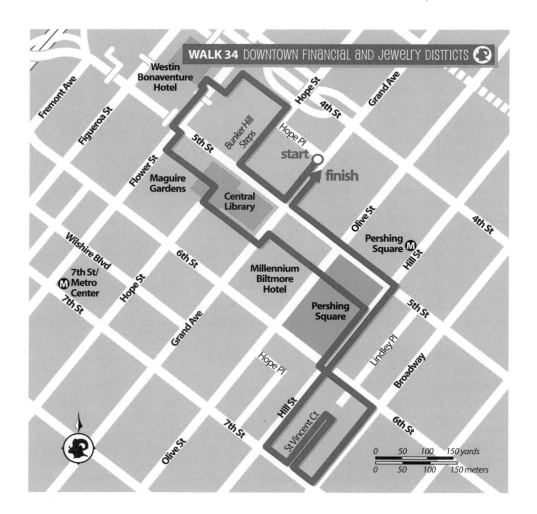

WALK 34 DOWNTOWN FINANCIAL AND JEWELRY DISTRICTS

Fremont Ave

Figueroa St

Westin
Bonaventure
Hotel

Hope St

Grand Ave

4th St

5th St

Bunker Hill
Steps

Hope Pl

Flower St

start

finish

Maguire
Gardens

Central
Library

Olive St

4th St

Wilshire Blvd

6th St

Pershing
Square M

Hill St

7th St/
M Metro
Center

Hope St

Millennium
Biltmore
Hotel

5th St

7th St

Grand Ave

Pershing
Square

Lindley Pl

Broadway

Hope Pl

Hill St

6th St

7th St

St Vincent Ct

0   50   100   150 yards

Olive St

0   50   100   150 meters

34 DOWNTOWN FINANCIAL AND JEWELRY DISTRICTS: MORE THAN MEETS THE EYE

BOUNDARIES: **Broadway, 4th St., Figueroa St., 7th St.**
THOMAS GUIDE COORDINATES: **Map 634; E4**
DISTANCE: **Approx. 1½ miles**
DIFFICULTY: **Moderate (includes stairways)**
PARKING: **Metered parking is available on Grand Ave., north of Hope Pl.**
NEAREST METRO STATION: **Pershing Square, Hill St. between 4th St. and 5th St. (Red Line)**

At first glance, downtown Los Angeles' financial district—with its anonymous mirrored-glass skyscrapers that could be from just about any modern metropolis—lacks much personality. But take some time to explore what's hidden among all those tall buildings, and you'll discover several of downtown's treasures, such as the innovative architecture of the Central Library, the extravagant interior of the Millennium Biltmore Hotel, and the thoughtfully designed Bunker Hill steps, as well as numerous public art projects. This walk also passes through the city's busy jewelry district, home to some of most beautiful movie palaces in the country.

● **Begin on Grand Ave. between Hope Pl. and 5th St. and head southwest, toward 5th St.**

● **Turn right on 5th St. The stately brick tower of the Millennium Biltmore Hotel rises on the southeast corner of Grand and 5th St. As you round the northwest corner, notice the classical Art Deco high-rise known as One Bunker Hill. This 14-story building, composed of solid limestone and buff-colored terra-cotta, once housed Southern California Edison.**

● **Turn right to ascend the gracefully curving Bunker Hill staircase. An elevated fountain built to resemble a stony brook runs down the center of the wide steps, which are also known as LA's own Spanish Steps. Look behind you to the other side of 5th St. to see the north entrance of the Central Library; an inscription carved into the stone façade reads, "Books alone are liberal and free: They give to all who ask. They emancipate all who serve them faithfully." As you make your way up the shallow steps, notice the cylindrical Library Tower reaching skyward on your right. The tallest** building in downtown LA, this distinctive landmark has been branded with the U.S. Bank logo on its lofty lighthouse, an unfortunate but inevitable sign of the times. The Citicorp building, or "*LA Law* building," is on your left.

● At the top of the steps is a small, circular plaza built around a fountain sculpture of a nude woman in bronze. McCormick & Schmick's, a sophisticated seafood restaurant and bar fashioned in dark wood, brass, and leather, is on the right. This is a popular haunt for the district's attorneys and bankers, who are lured by the bar's cheap and tasty happy hour food specials. Continue straight ahead onto Hope St., and notice the gleaming wings of Walt Disney Concert Hall several blocks to the north.

● When you reach the YMCA building on your left, just before 4th St., turn left to cut through the outdoor plaza. Various metal sculptures depicting male and female figures in athletic pursuits grace the patio.

● As you continue through the plaza, the mirrored glass cylindrical towers of the Westin Bonaventure Hotel loom ahead. Follow the first pedestrian walkway you encounter, and walk into the building. From there, descend the spiral stairway all the way down to the lobby. (Or, if you prefer, take a ride down in one of the building's famous glass elevators so that you can admire the view.) Built in 1978, the inside of the Bonaventure now appears dated, with lots of concrete and very little natural light. Once you've reached the lobby, exit the hotel through the glass doors on your left to Flower St.

● Turn right on Flower St. and then cross to the southeast corner of Flower St. and 5th St. so that you're on the same side as the Central Library.

● Follow the long, stepped walkway leading to the library's entrance, and admire the unique façade of the 1920s-era public building, which successfully incorporates elements of modern urban architecture with the ancient influence of Egyptian, Roman, Byzantine, and Islamic civilizations. The library's solitary tower is capped with a colorful, tiled pyramid depicting a sunburst and torch to represent the light of knowledge. A tiled reflecting pool runs down the center of the path leading up to the library entrance, and a lovely wall of spouting fountains lies in an alcove off to the right of the main entryway plaza. Cafe Pinot, an upscale restaurant serving California/French cuisine, is off to your left. The grassy public space and decorative fountains surrounding the library are known as the Maguire Gardens.

- Enter the library through the striking west-facing portal. Continue through the dark hallway into the main lobby, which is graced with a vibrantly painted ceiling. LA's Central Library is worth taking some time to explore; of particular architectural interest is the Tom Bradley Wing at the east end of the building, which consists of a dramatic, light-filled, eight-story atrium. You should also head upstairs to admire the Lodwrick M. Cook Rotunda, with its intricate, stenciled ceiling and enormous chandelier.

- After exploring the interior of the library, return to the main lobby on the first floor and leave the building through the southwest-facing exit (toward Hope St.).

- Once outside, descend the first two sets of stairs and then turn left to follow the sidewalk (do not descend the last set of stairs down to street level). On your right is the Hilton Checkers Hotel, a nicely restored 1920s building with ornate molded details.

- When you reach Grand Ave., carefully cross the street and then turn left. When you reach the valet parking area of the Millennium Biltmore Hotel, turn right to proceed to the hotel's rear entrance. This Beaux Arts landmark opened for business in 1923 and remains one of LA's finest classical hotels. The hotel's lobby is splendid, ornamented with a richly carved and painted ceiling, thick rugs, and distinguished furnishings.

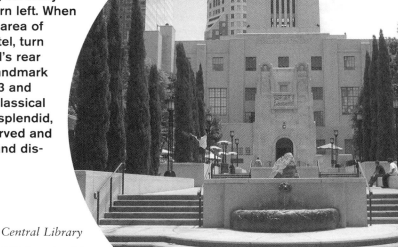

Central Library

● Continue straight through the lobby and then turn right into the building's grand hallway, which is lined with intricately carved stone pillars. Turn left at the elevators and descend the stairs into the front lobby. It doesn't seem possible, but this massive, high-ceilinged room—featuring an impressive, arched ceiling with an intricate, inlaid-wood design and a lovely central fountain—is even more magnificent than the first lobby you entered. Walk through the lobby to exit onto Olive St.

● Cross Olive St. to Pershing Square. Still considered a major downtown LA landmark, this public park has fallen hard from its former glory as a lush oasis in the center of the city. Today, this mostly concrete-paved space looks outdated, with its colorful geometric walls and sculptures, but it does afford a convenient raised clearing from which to survey the surrounding architecture. To the west is the distinguished brick façade of the Biltmore Hotel you just exited; immediately north of the Biltmore is the Gas Company Tower, a dramatic marble-and-steel high-rise, with a unique, curved, boat-like glass atrium at the very top. North of Pershing Square is the Art Deco-style Title Guarantee and Trust Building, which dates back to 1930. And if you look toward the southwest, you can catch a glimpse of the outdoor clock (colorfully

Back Story: What Ever Happened to Bunker Hill?

Founded in 1867, the region currently referred to as the Financial District sits atop Bunker Hill, a residential neighborhood that was leveled in the 1950s to make way for the skyscrapers that mark downtown Los Angeles today. Once a bustling residential community for Los Angeles professionals and their families, Bunker Hill degenerated over time and eventually became populated with unsavory rooming houses. In the 1960s, LA's Community Redevelopment Agency demolished what was left of the neighborhood's Victorian residences to make way for a "new downtown," complete with shiny skyscrapers, to signal the city's prosperity and status as an international commercial and banking center.

neon-lit at night) that overlooks the patio outside the Oviatt Building penthouse, another Art Deco landmark. At the south end of the park, a towering fountain that resembles a giant rain gutter spills a murky stream of water into a shallow, stone-lined pool.

- Cross Pershing Square to Hill St. and turn right.

- Turn left on 6th St. and walk for one block to Broadway. You're now in downtown's bustling and somewhat seedy Jewelry District.

- Turn right on Broadway. While the ornate French Baroque Los Angeles Theatre, at 615 S. Broadway, hasn't been an operational movie palace for many years, it's now available for filming and for private rentals. To visit the stunning interior of the theater, contact the Los Angeles Conservancy's Last Remaining Seats program at 213-623-2489.

Clifton's, one of LA's last surviving cafeteria-style restaurants, is located at 648 S. Broadway. The restaurant has been around since 1935, and while the food itself is nothing special, it is absolutely worth stopping in for a meal or a piece of pie so that you can marvel at the restaurant's throwback mountain-woods-themed interior.

- Turn right on 7th St. and walk to St. Vincent's Ct. on your right.

- Turn right to explore this unique and charming alley, which features a collection of Middle Eastern restaurants and bakeries housed behind Parisian cafe-style facades. Retrace your steps to 7th St.

View of skyscrapers from Pershing Square

- Turn right on 7th, and then turn right on Hill St., walking for two blocks.

- Turn left on 5th St. and continue for two more blocks, passing between the towering edifices of the Biltmore Hotel and the Gas Company Tower.

- Turn right on Grand Ave. to return to your starting point.

POINTS OF INTEREST

McCormick & Schmick's 633 W. 5th St., Los Angeles, CA 90071, 213-629-1929

Westin Bonaventure Hotel 404 S. Figueroa St., Los Angeles, CA 90071, 213-612-4743

Cafe Pinot 700 W. 5th St., Los Angeles, CA 90071, 213-239-6500

Central Library 630 W. 5th St., Los Angeles, CA 90071, 213-228-7000

Millennium Biltmore Hotel 506 S. Grand Ave., Los Angeles, CA 90071, 213-624-1011

Los Angeles Theatre 615 S. Broadway, Los Angeles CA 90014, 213-629-2939

Clifton's 648 S. Broadway, Los Angeles, CA 90014, 213-627-1673

route summary

1. Begin on Grand Ave. between Hope Pl. and 5th St. and head south toward 5th St.
2. Turn right on 5th St.
3. Ascend the Bunker Hill steps on your right.
4. At the top of the steps, continue straight ahead onto Hope St.
5. When you reach the YMCA building on your left, just before 4th St., turn left to cut through the outdoor plaza.
6. Follow the first pedestrian walkway into the Westin Bonaventure Hotel and then descend the spiral stairway to the lobby. Exit the hotel through the glass doors on your left to Flower St.
7. Turn right on Flower St. and then cross to the southeast corner of Flower St. and 5th St.
8. Follow the walkway to the entrance of the Central Library.
9. Pass through the library's entrance and continue through the dark hallway into the main lobby. Explore the interior of the library, including the upstairs rotunda and the eastern Bradley Wing.
10. Return to the main lobby on the first floor and leave the building through the southwest-facing exit (toward Hope St.).
11. Descend the first two sets of stairs and then turn left to follow the sidewalk (do not descend the last set of stairs down to street level).
12. Cross Grand Ave. and turn left.
13. When you reach the valet parking area of the Millennium Biltmore Hotel, turn right to proceed to the hotel's rear entrance.
14. Continue straight through the lobby and then turn right into the building's grand hallway. Turn left at the elevators and descend the stairs down into the front lobby. Walk through the lobby to exit onto Olive St.
15. Cross Olive St. to enter Pershing Square.
16. Cross Pershing Square to Hill St. and turn right.
17. Turn left on 6th St.
18. Turn right on Broadway.
19. Turn right on 7th St.
20. Turn right on St. Vincent's Ct., and then retrace your steps to 7th and turn right.
21. Turn right on Hill St.
22. Turn left on 5th St.
23. Turn right on Grand Ave. to return to your starting point.

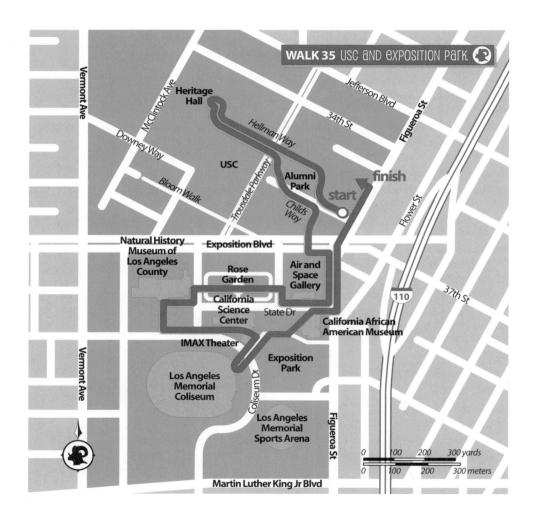

Vermont Ave

McClintock Ave

Heritage Hall

Downey Way

Hellman Way

Jefferson Blvd

34th St

Figueroa St

USC

Bloom Walk

Trousdale Parkway

Alumni Park

finish

start

Childs Way

Flower St

Natural History Museum of Los Angeles County

Exposition Blvd

Rose Garden

Air and Space Gallery

37th St

110

California Science Center

State Dr

California African American Museum

IMAX Theater

Exposition Park

Los Angeles Memorial Coliseum

Coliseum Dr

Los Angeles Memorial Sports Arena

Vermont Ave

Figueroa St

0   100   200   300 yards
0   100   200   300 meters

Martin Luther King Jr Blvd

35 USC aND EXPOSITION ParK: HIGHER LearNING

BOUNDARIES: **Figueroa St., Jefferson Blvd., Vermont Ave., Martin Luther King Jr. Blvd.**
THOMAS GUIDE COORDINATES: **Map 634; B1**
DISTANCE: **Approx. 1½ miles**
DIFFICULTY: **Easy (includes short flights of steps)**
PARKING: **Metered parking is available on Exposition Blvd. (The Expo Line will include a stop near this route, but the first phase isn't planned for completion until 2010.)**

The University of Southern California is a world-renowned private learning institution with a state-of-the-art campus, where students are extremely well cared for, and at the same time held to very high expectations. The attractive college grounds are located south of downtown Los Angeles. Just across the street is Exposition Park, a university-owned property that is home to numerous museums and outdoor educational displays, the classically inspired Los Angeles Memorial Coliseum, and a magnificent rose garden (open all year, except during pruning in January and February).

● Start on the west side of Figueroa St. at the intersection with Childs Way (just north of Exposition Blvd.). This is one of the entrances to the USC campus. Trojan Residence Hall and the admissions office are located at 615 Childs Way. Walk west on Childs Way. At 635 is the Alumni House, a simple but elegant white clap-board building dedicated in 1880 as the original University of Southern California. According to the plaque in front of the structure, this is the oldest university building in all of Southern California.

● Turn right to cut diagonally across the Alumni House plaza, heading northwest toward McCarthy Quad. You emerge into the expansive lawn area, where students gather to lounge around in the sun or frantically complete assignments on their laptops (the entire campus is equipped with wireless internet access). The quad is bordered to the north by Leavey Library, and by Doheny Library to the south—you can see the top of the Shrine Auditorium just beyond Leavey on the other side of Jefferson Blvd.

- Turn left, heading west, with Doheny Library on your left and the quad on your right. Continue straight along Hellman Way. Pass Alumni Park on your left before coming to the very collegiate-looking (even by USC architectural standards) Bovard Administration Building. As you pass the north side of the building, you can even peek into university president's opulent office, which occupies the northwest corner of the first floor. Next, you pass the renowned Annenberg School for Communication on your right and the Physical Education Building on your left.

- Turn right just past the Annenberg Building, and then turn left to enter Heritage Hall. In the lobby, you can admire every sports trophy USC has ever won, including countless Heisman trophies awarded to the Trojan football team. Quite impressive, if you're into that sort of thing.

- Exit Heritage Hall and retrace your steps back along Hellman Way past Bovard before turning right to cut diagonally across Alumni Park (heading southeast). Stop in the center of the park to admire the graceful Prentiss Memorial Fountain, entitled the "Four Corner Stones of American Democracy." You'll have to circle the fountain to discover each of these cornerstone values; the words are engraved into the fountain and illustrated by pretty little statues.

- Once through the park, turn left to head east on Childs Way. On your right, pass the Alfred Newman Recital Hall, which is decorated with an elaborate bas-relief of prehistoric mammals, and Hubbard Hall.

- Turn right just past the entrance to Lewis Hall, following the brick-paved passageway south toward Exposition Blvd.

- Exit through the gate onto Exposition Blvd. and cross the street at the crosswalk before turning left toward Figueroa St.

- Turn right on Figueroa and continue to State Dr., where you'll turn right to enter Exposition Park. Suspended on your right is an old United Airlines jet—one of the Aerospace Museum's several outdoor air/spacecraft displays.

- As you continue west on State Dr., you pass the Aerospace Museum, which was designed by Frank Gehry in 1984.

- Turn right just past the Aerospace Museum, passing the red brick façade of the old Armory building, which is now home to the California Science Center's Annenberg wing.

- Exposition Park's spectacular rose garden is on your left. Pause to admire the carefully ordered plots of colorful rosebushes, with the ornate, domed building of the original Los Angeles County Historical and Art Museum (now the east wing of the Natural History Museum) forming a picture-perfect backdrop. Walk through the garden toward the museum, breathing deeply to enjoy the sweetly scented air.

- Emerge from the garden and turn left, and then turn right at the next footpath, which you follow to the imposing entrance of the Natural History Museum. You can explore the grand interior architecture and educational displays of the museum for a moderate fee, or just continue on your walk to the California Science Center, which offers free admission.

- Turn left to follow the path leading south, away from the museum entrance, toward the Los Angeles Memorial Coliseum.

- Turn left at the next path and follow the walkway up into the remarkable plaza of the California Science Center. This area is covered by a huge, cylindrical metal structure, from which strings of gold balls hang down. The scientific premise of this contraption is dubious, but it's

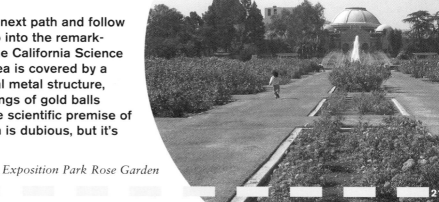

Exposition Park Rose Garden

fun to look at and provides a shady place to sit. Admission to the Science Center's permanent exhibit galleries is free, so take some time to explore this truly educational *and* entertaining museum. The IMAX Theater is next door—if you have an extra hour or two and around eight bucks to spend, watching a film on one of the enormous screens is a sensory treat. After exploring the California Science Center, exit back out into the plaza and turn left (heading in the opposite direction of the Natural History Museum).

- Just before you reach the parking structure adjacent to the IMAX Theater, turn right to follow the sidewalk, cross Coliseum Dr., and then turn left on the other side of the street to head toward the main entrance of the Coliseum. This 92,516-seat stadium held its first football game (USC versus Pomona College) in 1923 and has since hosted two Olympiads, two Super Bowls, and a World Series. Stop to check out the headless, anatomically correct statues of a male and female Olympians in front of the stadium entrance.

- Cross Coliseum Dr. once again to head back toward the parking structure, and then descend the staircase that leads into the sunken garden to the left of the structure.

- Follow the pleasant path past educational displays about hummingbirds and butterflies. An interactive exhibit on the top level of the parking structure shows kids how to use a lever to lift up an actual pickup truck—pretty cool. Continue to follow the path around the structure as it turns to the right, passing under an A-12 Blackbird spy craft, built in the 1960s.

- Ascend the stairs on your left and continue straight ahead, passing in front of the entrance to the California African American Museum. If the museum's open, take advantage of the free admission to learn more about the cultural and artistic contributions that African-Americans have made, particularly in California and the West.

- When you find yourself back at the jet exhibit at the intersection of State Dr. and Figueroa St., exit Exposition Park onto Figueroa and turn left. Ahead, you'll see the giant neon sign for Felix Chevrolet/Cadillac, a pop culture landmark graced with the likeness of the lovable cartoon cat himself.

● **If you parked your car on Exposition Blvd., turn left there, or continue on Figueroa St. to the start of the walk at the intersection of Childs Way.**

POINTS OF INTEREST

Exposition Park Rose Garden 701 State Dr., Los Angeles, CA 90037, 213-763-0114

Natural History Museum 900 Exposition Blvd., Los Angeles, CA 90007, 213-763-3466

California Science Center 700 State Dr., Los Angeles, CA 90037, 323-724-3623, 213-744-7400 (for IMAX Theater)

Los Angeles Memorial Coliseum 3911 S. Figueroa St., Los Angeles, CA 90037, 213-747-7111

California African American Museum 600 State Dr., Los Angeles, CA 90037, 213-744-7432

route summary

1. Start on the west side of Figueroa St. at the intersection with Childs Way (just north of Exposition Blvd.) and head west on Childs.

2. Turn right at the Alumni House and cut diagonally across the Alumni House plaza, heading northwest toward McCarthy Quad.

3. Turn left, heading west on Hellman Way.

4. Turn right just past the Annenberg Building, and then turn left to enter Heritage Hall.

5. Exit Heritage Hall and retrace your steps back along Hellman Way.

6. Turn right to cut diagonally across Alumni Park (heading southeast).

7. Once through the park, turn left to head east on Childs Way.

8. Turn right just past the entrance to Lewis Hall, heading south toward Exposition Blvd.

9. Exit through the gate onto Exposition Blvd. and cross the street at the crosswalk before turning left toward Figueroa St.

10. Turn right on Figueroa.

11. Turn right on State Dr. to enter Exposition Park.

12. Turn right just pass the Aerospace Museum, passing the red brick façade of the old Armory building.

13. Enter the Exposition Park Rose Garden on your left and walk the length of the garden.

14. Emerge from the garden and turn left, and then turn right at the next footpath, heading toward the main entrance of the Natural History Museum.

15. Turn left to follow the path leading south away from the museum entrance toward the Los Angeles Memorial Coliseum.

16. Turn left at the next path and follow the walkway up into the plaza of the California Science Center.

17. Just before you reach the parking structure adjacent to the IMAX Theater, turn right to follow the sidewalk, cross Coliseum Dr., and then turn left on the other side of the street to head toward the main entrance of the Coliseum.

18. Cross the Coliseum Dr. once again toward the parking structure and then descend the staircase that leads down into the sunken garden to the left of the structure.

19. Follow the garden path adjacent to the parking structure, continuing along the sidewalk as it turns to the right.

20. Ascend the stairs on your left and continue straight ahead, passing the entrance to the California African American Museum.

21. When you reach the intersection of State Dr. and Figueroa St., exit Exposition Park onto Figueroa and turn left.

22. If you parked on Exposition Blvd., turn left there to return to your parked car, or continue on Figueroa to your starting point at the intersection of Childs Way.

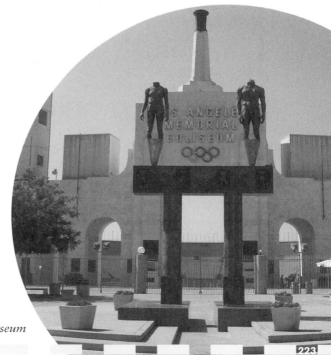

Los Angeles Memorial Coliseum

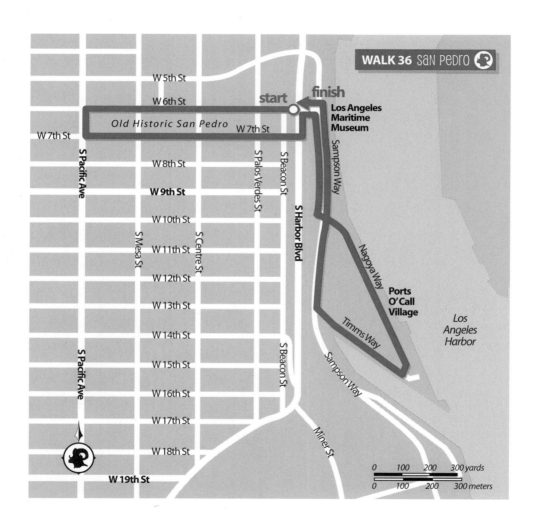

W 5th St

W 6th St

start

finish

Los Angeles
Maritime
Museum

Old Historic San Pedro

W 7th St

W 7th St

W 8th St

S Pacific Ave

S Palos Verdes St

S Beacon St

Sampson Way

W 9th St

W 10th St

W 11th St

S Mesa St

S Centre St

W 12th St

W 13th St

Nagoya Way

Ports
O'Call
Village

Los
Angeles
Harbor

W 14th St

Timms Way

W 15th St

S Beacon St

W 16th St

Sampson Way

W 17th St

W 18th St

S Pacific Ave

Miner St

W 19th St

0	100	200	300 yards
0	100	200	300 meters

36 san pedro: make way for gentrification

BOUNDARIES: **Pacific Ave., Los Angeles Harbor, 5th St., 16th St.**
THOMAS GUIDE COORDINATES: **Map 824; C5**
DISTANCE: **Approx. 2 miles**
DIFFICULTY: **Easy**
PARKING: **Free parking is available in the lot for the Los Angeles Maritime Museum.**

Due in large part to its coveted waterfront location and mild climate, the city of San Pedro is ripe for gentrification. This port city's ambitious "From Bridge to Breakwater" revitalization and redevelopment plan includes an extension of the picturesque waterfront promenade, commercial and residential development in downtown San Pedro, and improvement of the city's public transportation. Your best bet for visiting downtown San Pedro is during a "First Thursday" celebration, which features gallery openings, street vendors, and entertainment between 6 P.M. and 9 P.M. on the first Thursday of each month.

● **Begin at the corner of 6th St. and Harbor Blvd. in the parking lot for the Los Angeles Maritime Museum and the Downtown/6th St. stop for San Pedro's waterfront Red Car line. This vintage electric trolley runs on the weekends and uses replica railcars patterned after the 1909 Pacific Electric cars to take visitors between the World Cruise Center north of downtown and the Ports O' Call Village to the south. The $1 trolley fare also includes free transfers to the rubber-tired trolley line that heads as far south as Cabrillo Beach and the Cabrillo Marine Aquarium.**

Take some time to explore the historic artifacts displayed in front of the Maritime Museum, including a ship's anchor and steering wheel, a memorial propeller from a WWII warship, and the front of the hull of the U.S.S. *Los Angeles*. If you have a few dollars and some extra time to spend, you can explore the museum itself, which boasts an impressive collection of ships, models, and navigational equipment, as well as rotating exhibits.

At the corner of Harbor and 6th St. is the American Merchant Marine Veterans Memorial, which consists of a beautiful fountain sculpture by Jasper D'Ambrosi that depicts one man rescuing another from the sea.

- Follow 6th St. west toward Old Historic San Pedro. The sidewalk on both sides of the street is lined with plaques for athletes and sports professionals who have some connection with either San Pedro or Los Angeles.

- After crossing Centre St., 6th St. becomes trendier, featuring an assortment of boutiques, bistros, and breweries, as well as more established businesses and art galleries housed in historic storefronts. One such shop, Williams Book Store (established in 1909), is worth stopping in to browse the books and magazines and get a dose of San Pedro history from the proprietor.

  The Art Deco Warner Grand Theatre is located at 478 W. 6th St. The theater opened in 1931 and is on the National Register of Historic Places; today it serves as a venue for shows, concerts, and classic films.

- Turn left on Pacific Ave. and walk one block.

- Turn left on 7th St. to enter the heart of the Downtown San Pedro Arts District, which features more galleries, shops, and eateries. This area also includes the inevitable upscale loft developments that show up in any burgeoning artists' community. The Bank Lofts in the historical Bank of San Pedro building are located at the corner of Mesa St. Continue on 7th St. all the way back to Harbor Blvd.

- Turn left on Harbor Blvd.

- Turn right on 6th St., where you will pass your starting point in front of the Maritime Museum.

- Instead of stopping, continue on 6th to Sampson Way and turn right. Follow the road along the harbor front, passing the restaurant Acapulco before coming to Fisherman's Seafood, at 950 Sampson Way. This festive restaurant, with its huge outdoor patio, marks the beginning of Ports O' Call Village, a collection of restaurants, fish markets, and specialty stops designed to resemble a New England seaside village with cobblestone streets and quaint storefronts.

- Bear left onto Nagoya Way to continue toward Ports O' Call. It has the feel of a tourist trap, but it appears to be popular with locals as well, thanks to the staggering selection of fresh fish and tempting deep-fried delicacies. You might want to grab a bite at one of the tables overlooking the harbor, where you can wave to the departing cruise ships.

● After walking the length of Ports O' Call Village, cut across the parking lot on the right and return via Timms Way, which merges with Sampson Way. At the intersection with Sampson Way is Utros Cafe, another festive-looking seafood restaurant located on Fisherman's Wharf.

● Another Red Car trolley station is located just across the street on Sampson Way. If you'd like to give your feet a rest and check out the beautiful replica antique railcar, you can board and get a ride directly back to your starting point at the Downtown/6th St. stop. If you'd rather hoof it, turn right on Sampson Way and follow it back to the intersection of 6th St.

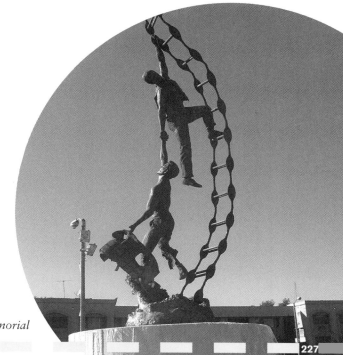

American Merchant Marine Veterans Memorial

POINTS OF INTEREST

Los Angeles Maritime Museum Berth 84 (foot of 6th St.), San Pedro, CA 90731, 310-548-7618

Williams Book Store 443 W. 6th St., San Pedro, CA 90731, 310-832-3631

Warner Grand Theatre 478 W. 6th St., San Pedro, CA 90731, 310-548-7672

Acapulco 750 Sampson Way, San Pedro, CA 90731, 310-548-6800

Fisherman's Seafood 950 Sampson Way, San Pedro, CA 90731, 310-519-7333

Utros Cafe Berth 73, San Pedro, CA 90731, 310-547-5022

route summary

1. Begin at the corner of 6th St. and Harbor Blvd. and follow 6th west toward Old Historic San Pedro.
2. Turn left on Pacific Ave.
3. Turn left on 7th St.
4. Turn left on Harbor Blvd.
5. Turn right back onto 6th St.
6. Turn right on Sampson Way.
7. Bear left onto Nagoya Way.
8. Cut across the Ports O' Call Village parking lot on the right and return via Timms Way, which merges with Sampson Way.
9. Either turn right on Sampson Way to return to your starting point at the intersection of 6th St., or take the trolley back to the Downtown/6th St. stop.

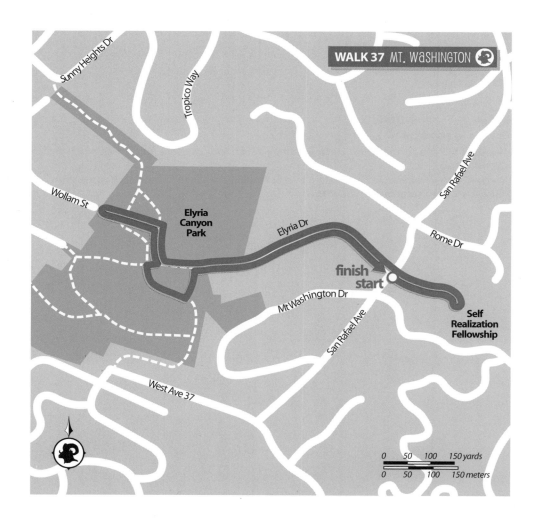

WALK 37 MT. WASHINGTON

Sunny Heights Dr

Tropico Way

San Rafael Ave

Rome Dr

Wollam St

Elyria
Canyon
Park

Elyria Dr

finish
start

Mt Washington Dr

San Rafael Ave

Self
Realization
Fellowship

West Ave 37

0   50   100   150 yards
0   50   100   150 meters

37 MT. WASHINGTON: Far From The City In Spirit

DIRECTIONS: **This route starts at the peak of Mt. Washington, which can be tough to find. Follow these driving directions in order to successfully navigate the twists and turns of the narrow canyon roads:**
- **Begin at the intersection of Figueroa Ave. and Marmion Way.**
- **Head north on Marmion Way.**
- **Turn left on Ave. 45.**
- **Turn right on Cañon Crest Dr.**
- **Turn left on Ave. 46.**
- **Turn left on Rome Dr.**
- **Turn left on San Rafael Ave.**
- **Arrive at the intersection with Elyria Dr.**

THOMAS GUIDE COORDINATES: **Map 594; J4**
DISTANCE: **¼ mile to 1½ miles, depending on route chosen**
DIFFICULTY: **Easy to strenuous (includes short flights of steps and optional dirt hiking trail)**
PARKING: **Free parking is available just inside the gates of the Self-Realization Fellowship grounds.**

Mt. Washington is one of several idyllic communities hidden in the hills between downtown Los Angeles and Pasadena. This rustic neighborhood is populated with a collection of artistic, laid-back, nature-loving individuals, so it's no surprise that it is also home to the world headquarters of the Self-Realization Fellowship. Founded in 1920 by Paramahansa Yogananda, this worldwide religious organization seeks to bring together people of all creeds in the pursuit of world peace and harmony—a noble goal, to be sure.

This walk can be whatever you make of it—either a short stroll through the grounds of the fellowship, where you can meditate on the beauty of your serene surroundings atop the hill and enjoy panoramic views of the city below, or a genuine hike that takes you from these carefully manicured grounds down through the rustic beauty of nearby Elyria Canyon Park and back up again.

● **Begin just inside the gates of the Self-Realization Fellowship International Headquarters at the intersection of San Rafael Ave. and Elyria Dr. A small visitor's** center is just inside the gate to your left—here you can speak to a volunteer or browse through literature to learn more about this popular pan-religious movement.

- Head into the fellowship grounds, passing a large lawn area on your right before you come to a tennis court. Descend the steps and cut lengthwise across the court. To your right is a sundial surrounding by benches—from here, you can sit and enjoy a view of the downtown high-rises a few miles south of Mt. Washington.

- Continue along the gravel path, which leads through a lush garden of ferns, ficus trees, and palms. Private alcoves set back into the vegetation on either side of the path offer a place to contemplate or meditate; you will be serenaded by the sound of a trickling fountain. Eventually, you come to a table and chairs carved out of stone that sit beneath a stand of pine trees—another lovely spot to stop for a rest, engage in deep thought, or stop thinking altogether.

- Follow the path past the stone table and chairs as it turns to the left, and ascend a short flight of steps. Pass a planter filled with water and lily pads, and continue up the next set of steps, passing through a rose garden before you emerge back into the paved parking area.

- Turn around here to head back toward the entrance to the fellowship. On your right is the main building, a distinctive, three-story, flat-roofed structure established as the Mt. Washington Inn, a popular resort for Hollywood stars and society types in the late 1800s and early years of the 20th century. The Mt. Washington Development Company even built a short railway leading up and down the hill to get patrons to and from the inn. The railway has long since shut down, but the former passenger depot is still standing, down the hill at the corner of Ave. 43 and Marmion Way.

  After passing the former hotel, you reach a small gazebo on your right. Inside is a wishing well decorated with peaceful greetings and wishes from Paramahansa Yogananda himself.

- At this point, you can return to your car and end the walk, or you could opt for a real workout by continuing on the route that follows into Elyria Canyon Park, which is located down the street from the Self-Realization Fellowship.

Addendum:

- Exit the fellowship grounds and continue west on Elyria Dr., crossing San Rafael Ave. A stunning, shingled Craftsman sits on the corner on your right.

- Follow the road as it turns to the left. You can see the chaparral-covered hills of Elyria Canyon sloping down on your right. Continue all the way to the end of the street, where you arrive at a trailhead.

- Follow the trail as it starts to descend through the grassy meadowland into the canyon. Thirty-five-acre Elyria Canyon Park, part of the Santa Monica Mountains Conservancy parkland, is home to one of the last remaining stands of California black walnut in the greater Los Angeles area. If you've brought your dog along for the hike, be sure to keep him on-leash in the park. You should also watch out for poison oak, although you should be safe as long as you stick to the clearly marked trails.

- When you come to the first split in the trail, take the right-hand path, which affords a view of Glendale in the distance.

- At the next split, continue to follow your path as it curves to the right. The trail widens slightly here and shows remnants of asphalt paving. Continue downhill along the shady trail.

- At the next split in the trail, follow the path that curves downhill to your left a short distance to the floor of the canyon and the Elyria Canyon Park entrance at Wollam St.

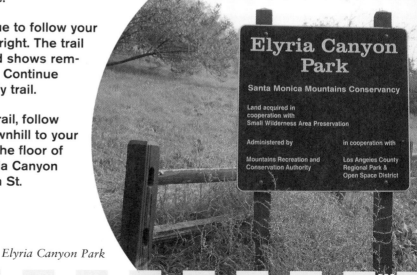

Elyria Canyon Park

- Head back up the trail, bearing right at the split to continue along the same path you took down.

- When you return to the point where the path widens, take the narrow dirt trail that branches off to the right (instead of continuing back up the same trail you followed into the park). Follow the new trail as it curves to the left, affording a view of the other side of the canyon and the large homes perched high on the ridge above.

- At the next split, take the narrow trail to the left that heads uphill and curves around through the bushes, past a bench and trash can, before it reconnects with your original path.

- Turn right and take the trail back up to your starting point at the end of Elyria Dr.

- Follow Elyria Dr. back to the entrance of the Self-Realization Fellowship, where you began.

POINT OF INTEREST

Self-Realization Fellowship 3880 San Rafael Dr., Los Angeles, CA 90065, 323-225-2471

route summary

1. Begin at the entrance to the Self-Realization Fellowship at the intersection of San Rafael Ave. and Elyria Dr.
2. Head into the fellowship grounds, and then descend the stairs into the tennis court on your right. Cut lengthwise across the court.
3. Follow the gravel path through the garden.
4. Continue to follow the path as it turns to the left, and then continue up the steps, eventually ending at the parking lot.
5. Return to your starting point just inside the entrance.

Addendum:

6. Exit the gates of the Self-Realization Fellowship and continue west on Elyria Dr.
7. Follow the road as it turns to the left and continue all the way to the street's end.
8. Follow the dirt hiking trail into Elyria Canyon Park.
9. When you come to the first split in the trail, take the right-hand path.
10. At the next split, continue to follow your path as it curves to the right and continues downhill.
11. At the next split in the trail, take the path that curves downhill to your left, and follow it to the park entrance at Wollam St.
12. Head back up the trail, bearing right at the split to continue along the same path you took down.
13. When you return to the point where the path widens, take the narrow dirt trail that branches off to the right and follow the trail as it curves to the left.
14. At the next split, take the narrow trail to the left that heads uphill back to the point where it reconnects with your original path.
15. Turn right and take the trail back up to your starting point at the end of Elyria Dr.
16. Follow Elyria Dr. back to the entrance of the Self-Realization Fellowship, where you began.

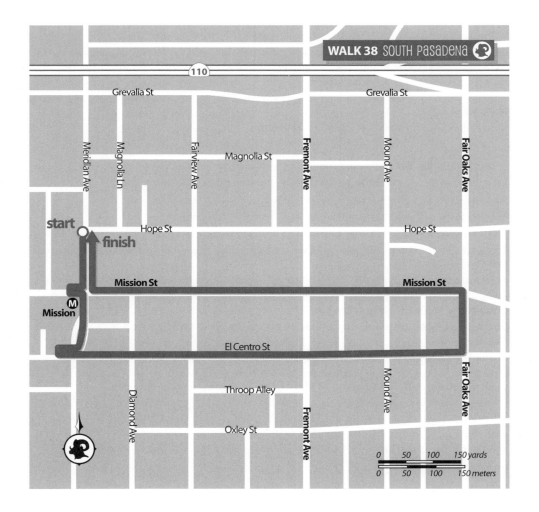

WALK 38 SOUTH PASADENA

110

Grevalia St

Grevalia St

Meridian Ave

Magnolia Ln

Fairview Ave

Magnolia St

Fremont Ave

Mound Ave

Fair Oaks Ave

start

finish

Hope St

Hope St

Mission St

Mission St

M
Mission

El Centro St

Diamond Ave

Throop Alley

Mound Ave

Fair Oaks Ave

Oxley St

Fremont Ave

0   50   100   150 yards

0   50   100   150 meters

38 SOUTH PASADENA: A HIPPER MAYBERRY

BOUNDARIES: **Fair Oaks Ave., 110 Freeway, Orange Grove Ave., El Centro St.**
THOMAS GUIDE COORDINATES: **Map 595; G2**
DISTANCE: **Approx. 1 mile**
DIFFICULTY: **Easy**
PARKING: **Free street parking is available on Meridian Ave., and there is a public parking structure on the corner of Meridian and Mission St.**
NEAREST METRO STATION: **Mission St. and Meridian Ave. (Gold Line)**

One local store proprietor refers to South Pasadena as a "hipper Mayberry," and the description is apt. This city has a lovely, small-town sense of community, but at the same time it is fast becoming a happening shopping and dining destination. This walk begins at the hub of South Pas: Mission Meridian Village, an urban village centered around the Metro Gold Line station to reduce traffic and develop a community center by building housing within close proximity to public transportation and commercial attractions. Development around public transit hubs has become a popular trend in Los Angeles within the last few years, but the execution seems more successful in South Pasadena than elsewhere.

● Begin at the corner of Hope St. and Meridian Ave. The Mission Meridian complex's immaculate Craftsman duplexes line the west side of Meridian. Head south on Meridian, passing a boutique, a florist, and a public parking structure. Heirloom Bakery & Cafe, at 807 Meridian Ave., will no doubt tempt you with its scrumptious selection of goodies.

Buster's, "the coffee stop by the tracks," sits on the northeast corner of Mission and Meridian. The cheerfully painted java house—a popular neighborhood spot for more than 20 years—slings a selection of organic brews, iced drinks, and Fosselman's ice cream. Across the street, on the northwest corner, is 750 ml wine bar, which is housed in the former Mission Arroyo Hotel building, a South Pasadena Cultural Landmark.

● When you reach Mission St., turn right to visit Organic Rush, which sells environmentally friendly bath, home, and baby products, at 962 Mission St.

- Cross to the south side of Mission St. at the crosswalk and turn around to head east on Mission, toward the Metro station.

- Turn right back onto Meridian. Pass a large, woven metal sculpture depicting, appropriately enough, a man walking. The South Pasadena Historical Museum, located inside the Meridian Iron Works building at 913 Meridian, features exhibits depicting South Pasadena's history, beginning with the original Native American residents, along with photos of the city during its early years of development. It's free to the public, so why not pop in and check it out? It's also worthwhile to cross to the island in the middle of the street to check out another cultural landmark, the Watering Trough and Wayside Station, which was erected in 1906 as a rest stop for horses and their riders. On the corner of Meridian and El Centro St. is Bistro de la Gare, a charming French restaurant and wine bar.

- Turn right on El Centro to visit Nicole's Gourmet Foods, a plant nursery, and the Los Angeles-bound platform for the South Pasadena Gold Line station.

- Turn around to retrace your steps back to Meridian, and then continue east on El Centro. At 1009 El Centro is Firefly Bistro, another charming restaurant with a vine-covered entrance and welcoming patio. It's obvious that South Pasadena diners very much enjoy a tasty meal al fresco accompanied by a carefully matched glass of wine, but then, who doesn't?

  At 1019 El Centro, you pass the South Pasadena Bank Building, another cultural landmark; the two-story brick building now houses a hair salon and a coffee shop (South Pas dwellers appear to love their java, as well).

  After crossing Diamond Ave. you come to the South Pasadena Library Community Room, a distinguished brick and stone building set in a small, shady park. The city's Unified School District Administration building is on the opposite side of the street. (South Pasadena is known to lure young families away from the city of Los Angeles with its excellent school system.)

  Continue on El Centro all the way to Fair Oaks Ave., passing apartment buildings, the Fremont Centre Theatre, and a culinary arts school.

- Turn left on Fair Oaks Ave.

- At the light, cross to the north side of Mission St. and turn left. At 1526 Mission, Fair Oaks Pharmacy and Soda Fountain, originally opened in 1915, offers a heavy dose of nostalgia with its tin ceilings, honeycomb-tile floors, and old-fashioned soda fountain. Stop in for a hand-dipped malt, egg cream, or lime rickey, and imagine what it was like when this served as a popular Route 66 pit stop.

  At 1510 Mission, you reach Dinosaur Farm, a toy store with a delightfully back-to-basics vibe that sells a terrific assortment of craft kits, musical instruments, games, and more. The store also offers story time and kids' classes in the back room.

  As you continue west on Mission, you pass more clothing and home interiors boutiques, antique shops, and other independent businesses; major chains are refreshingly few and far between in this part of town. Noteworthy stores include Livin' Art, at 1130 Mission; Book 'Em Mysteries, at 1118; and Mission Wines, at 1114.

  At 1040 Mission, Mike & Anne's offers delicious seasonal dishes with a gourmet flair on a welcoming patio. Knitting and needlepoint shop Abuelita's is at 1012. Across the street are Mission Street Yoga and Puff, a cheerful beauty-supply store selling hard-to-find boutique brands and offering custom facial treatments.

- When you reach Meridian Ave., turn right to return to your starting point at the corner of Hope St.

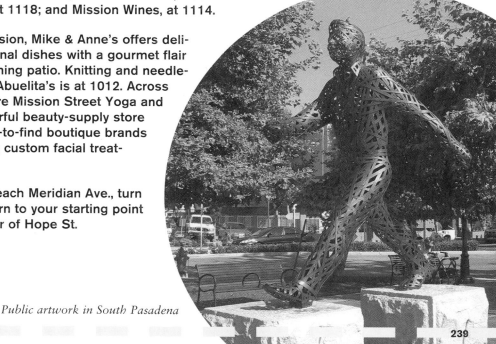

Public artwork in South Pasadena

POINTS OF INTEREST

Heirloom Bakery & Cafe 807 Meridian Ave., South Pasadena, CA 91030, 626-441-0042

Buster's 1006 Mission St., South Pasadena, CA 91030, 626-441-0744

750 ml 966 Mission St., South Pasadena, CA 91030, 626-799-0711

Organic Rush 960 Mission St., South Pasadena, CA 91030, 626-799-8099

South Pasadena Historical Museum 913 Meridian St., South Pasadena, CA 91030, 626-799-9089

Bistro de la Gare 921 Meridian Ave., South Pasadena, CA 91030, 626-799-8828

Nicole's Gourmet Foods 921 Meridian Ave. Ste. B, South Pasadena, CA 91030, 626-403-5751

Firefly Bistro 1009 El Centro St., South Pasadena, CA 91030, 626-441-2443

Fair Oaks Pharmacy and Soda Fountain 1526 Mission St., South Pasadena, CA 91030, 626-799-1414

Dinosaur Farm 1510 Mission St., South Pasadena, CA 91030, 626-441-2767

Livin' Art 1130 Mission St., South Pasadena, CA 91030, 626-799-8278

Book 'Em Mysteries 1118 Mission St., South Pasadena, CA 91030, 626-799-9600

Mission Wines 1114 Mission St., South Pasadena, CA 91030, 626-403-9463

Mike & Anne's 1040 Mission St., South Pasadena, CA 91030, 626-799-7199

Abuelita's 1012 Mission St., South Pasadena, CA 91030, 626-799-0355

Mission Street Yoga 1017 Mission St., South Pasadena, CA 91030, 626-441-1144

Puff 1005 Mission St., South Pasadena, CA 91030, 626-799-2864

route summary

1. Begin at the corner of Hope St. and Meridian Ave. and head south on Meridian.
2. Turn right on Mission St. to explore a couple of shops.
3. Cross to the south side of Mission St. and retrace your steps to Meridian.
4. Turn right on Meridian.
5. Turn right on El Centro St. to explore a restaurant and plant nursery.
6. Retrace your steps back to Meridian, and then continue east on El Centro.
7. Turn left on Fair Oaks Ave.
8. Cross Mission St. at the light and turn left on Mission.
9. Turn right on Meridian Ave. to return to your starting point at the corner of Hope St.

APPENDIX 1: WALKS BY THEME

PEOPLE WATCHING

Northwest Santa Monica (Walk 2)
Venice Beach (Walk 4)
Sunset Strip (Walk 12)
West Hollywood (Walk 13)
Miracle Mile (Walk 14)
Whitley Heights and Hollywood Boulevard
(Walk 17)
Larchmont Village and Windsor Square
(Walk 21)
West Silver Lake (Walk 27)

ARTS AND CULTURE

Southeast Santa Monica (Walk 3)
UCLA Campus (Walk 6)
Leimert Park Village (Walk 9)
NoHo Arts District (Walk 10)
Miracle Mile (Walk 14)
Brand Park and Kenneth Village (Walk 25)
El Pueblo de Los Angeles and Chinatown
(Walk 31)
Little Tokyo (Walk 32)
Downtown Civic Center (Walk 33)
Downtown Financial and Jewelry Districts
(Walk 34)
USC and Exposition Park (Walk 35)
San Pedro (Walk 36)

DINING, SHOPPING, AND ENTERTAINMENT

Northwest Santa Monica (Walk 2)
Venice Beach (Walk 4)
North Culver City (Walk 7)
Downtown Culver City (Walk 8)
Leimert Park Village (Walk 9)
NoHo Arts District (Walk 10)
Studio City's Woodbridge Park (Walk 11)
Sunset Strip (Walk 12)
West Hollywood (Walk 13)
Miracle Mile (Walk 14)
Larchmont Village and Windsor Square
(Walk 21)
Koreatown/Wilshire Center (Walk 22)
Atwater Village (Walk 26)
West Silver Lake (Walk 27)
El Pueblo de Los Angeles and Chinatown
(Walk 31)
Little Tokyo (Walk 32)
South Pasadena (Walk 38)

architectural tours

Mar Vista (Walk 5)
North Culver City (Walk 7)
Carthay Circle and South Carthay
   (Walk 15)
Melrose Hill (Walk 20)
Los Feliz (Walk 23)
East Silver Lake (Walk 28)
Echo Park and Angelino Heights
   (Walk 29)
Downtown Civic Center (Walk 33)
Downtown Financial and Jewelry Districts
   (Walk 34)

peaceful escapes

Castellammare (Walk 1)
High Tower and the Hollywood Bowl
   (Walk 16)
Lower Beachwood Canyon (Walk 18)
Upper Beachwood Canyon (Walk 19)
Franklin Hills (Walk 24)
Elysian Heights (Walk 30)
Mt. Washington (Walk 37)

serious workouts

Castellammare (Walk 1)
Northwest Santa Monica (Walk 2)
Downtown Culver City (Walk 8)
Sunset Strip (Walk 12)
Lower Beachwood Canyon (Walk 18)
Upper Beachwood Canyon (Walk 19)
Los Feliz (Walk 23)
East Silver Lake (Walk 28)
Echo Park and Angelino Heights (Walk 29)

APPENDIX 2: POINTS OF INTEREST

FOOD aND DrINK

101 Coffee Shop 6145 Franklin Ave., Los Angeles, CA 90028, 323-467-1175 *(WALK 18)*
750 ml 966 Mission St., South Pasadena, CA 91030, 626-799-0711 *(WALK 38)*
Abbot's Habit 1401 Abbot Kinney Blvd., Venice, CA 90291, 310-399-1171 *(WALK 4)*
Acapulco 750 Sampson Way, San Pedro, CA 90731, 310-548-6800 *(WALK 36)*
Alcove Cafe & Bakery 1929 Hillhurst Ave., Los Angeles, CA 90027, 323-644-0100 *(WALK 23)*
Alegria on Sunset 3510 W. Sunset Blvd., Los Angeles, CA 90026, 323-913-1422 *(WALK 27)*
Aroma Coffee and Tea Co. 4360 Tujunga Ave., Studio City, CA 91604, 818-508-6505 *(WALK 11)*
Asia 3179 Los Feliz Blvd., Los Angeles, CA 90039, 323-906-9498 *(WALK 26)*
Back Door Bakery and Cafe 1710 Silver Lake Blvd., Los Angeles, CA 90026, 323-662-7927 *(WALK 28)*
Back on Broadway 2024 Broadway Blvd., Santa Monica, CA 90404, 310-453-8919 *(WALK 3)*
Bank Heist 5303 Lankershim Blvd., North Hollywood, CA 91601, 818-760-1648 *(WALK 10)*
BCD Tofu House 3575 Wilshire Blvd., Los Angeles, CA 90010, 213-382-6677 *(WALK 22)*
Beachwood Market 2701 Belden Dr., Los Angeles, CA 90068, 323-464-7154 *(WALK 19)*
Beacon 3280 Helms Ave., Culver City, CA 90034, 310-838-7500 *(WALK 7)*
Bigfoot Lodge 3172 Los Feliz Blvd., Los Angeles, CA 90039, 323-662-9227 *(WALK 26)*
Birds 5925 Franklin Ave., Los Angeles, CA 90028, 323-465-0175 *(WALK 18)*
Bistro de la Gare 921 Meridian Ave., South Pasadena, CA 91030, 626-799-8828 *(WALK 38)*
Bizou Garden Bistro 2450 Colorado Ave., Santa Monica, CA 90404, 310-582-8203 *(WALK 3)*
BottleRock 3847 Main St., Culver City, CA 90232, 310-836-9463 *(WALK 8)*
Bourgeois Pig 5931 Franklin Ave., Los Angeles, CA 90028, 323-464-600 *(WALK 18)*
Buster's 1006 Mission St., South Pasadena, CA 91030, 626-441-0744 *(WALK 38)*
Cabo Cantina 8301 W. Sunset Blvd., West Hollywood, CA 90069, 323-822-7820 *(WALK 12)*
Cafe Boulangerie 804 Montana Ave., Santa Monica, CA 90403, 310-451-4998 *(WALK 2)*
Cafe du Village 139½ N. Larchmont Blvd., Los Angeles, CA 90004, 323-466-3996 *(WALK 21)*
Cafe Med 8615 W. Sunset Blvd., West Hollywood, CA 90069, 310-652-0445 *(WALK 12)*
Cafe Pinot 700 W 5th St., Los Angeles, CA 90071, 213-239-6500 *(WALK 34)*
Caffe Primo 8590 W. Sunset Blvd., West Hollywood, CA 90069, 310-289-8895 *(WALK 12)*
Caioti Pizza Cafe 4346 Tujunga Ave., Studio City, CA 91604, 818-761-3588 *(WALK 11)*

Carney's Restaurant 8351 W. Sunset Blvd., West Hollywood, CA 90069, 323-654-8300 *(WALK 12)*

Casa la Golondrina 17 Olvera St., Los Angeles, CA 90012, 213-628-4349 *(WALK 31)*

Chan Dara Restaurant 310 N. Larchmont Blvd., Los Angeles, CA 90004, 323-467-1052 *(WALK 21)*

Cheese Store of Silver Lake 3926 W. Sunset Blvd., Los Angeles, CA 90029, 323-644-7511 *(WALK 27)*

Clifton's 648 S. Broadway, Los Angeles, CA 90014, 213-627-1673 *(WALK 34)*

Club Tee Gee 3210 Glendale Blvd., Los Angeles, CA 90039, 323-669-9631 *(WALK 26)*

Culver City Farmers Market Main St. between Culver Blvd. and Venice Blvd., Culver City, CA 90230, Tuesdays 3 P.M. to 7 P.M. *(WALK 8)*

Dresden Restaurant 1760 N. Vermont Ave., Hollywood, CA 90027, 323-665-4294 *(WALK 23)*

Eat Well 3916 W. Sunset Blvd., Los Angeles, CA 90029, 323-664-1624 *(WALK 27)*

Eclectic Wine Bar & Grille 5156 Lankershim Blvd., North Hollywood, CA 91601, 818-760-2233 *(WALK 10)*

El Conquistador 3932 W. Sunset Blvd., Los Angeles, CA 90029, 323-666-0265 *(WALK 27)*

Electric Lotus 4656 Franklin Ave., Los Angeles, CA 90027, 323-953-0040 *(WALK 23)*

Erewhon Natural Foods Market 7660 Beverly Blvd., Los Angeles, CA 90036, 323-937-0777 *(WALK 14)*

Fair Oaks Pharmacy and Soda Fountain 1526 Mission St., South Pasadena, CA 91030, 626-799-1414 *(WALK 38)*

Famima!! 8525 Santa Monica Blvd., West Hollywood, CA 90069, 310-659-2684 *(WALK 13)*

Farmers Market 6333 W. 3rd St., Los Angeles, CA 90036, 323-933-9211 *(WALK 14)*

Firefly Bistro 1009 El Centro St., South Pasadena, CA 91030, 626-441-2443 *(WALK 38)*

Fisherman's Seafood 950 Sampson Way, San Pedro, CA 90731, 310-519-7333 *(WALK 36)*

Foo Chow 949 N. Hill St., Los Angeles, CA 90012, 213-485-1294 *(WALK 31)*

Ford's Filling Station 9531 Culver Blvd., Culver City, CA 90232, 310-202-1470 *(WALK 8)*

Fraiche 9411 Culver Blvd., Culver City, CA 90232, 310-839-6800 *(WALK 8)*

Fred 62 1850 N. Vermont Ave., Los Angeles, CA 90027, 323-667-0062 *(WALK 23)*

Good Microbrew and Grill 3725 W. Sunset Blvd., Los Angeles, CA 90029, 323-660-3645 *(WALK 27)*

Grand Casino Bakery 3826 Main St., Culver City, CA 90232, 310-202-6969 *(WALK 8)*

Grand Central Market 317 S. Broadway, Los Angeles, CA 90012, 213-624-2378 *(WALK 33)*

Heirloom Bakery & Cafe 807 Meridian Ave., South Pasadena, CA 91030, 626-441-0042 *(WALK 38)*

Home 1760 Hillhurst Ave., Los Angeles, CA 90027, 323-669-0211 *(WALK 23)*

Hop Louie 950 Mei Ling Way (inside Central Plaza), Los Angeles, CA 90012, 213-628-4244 *(WALK 31)*

House of Pies 1869 N. Vermont Ave., Los Angeles, CA 90027, 323-666-9961 *(WALK 23)*

Il Sole 8741 W. Sunset Blvd., West Hollywood, CA 90069, 310-657-1182 *(WALK 12)*

India Sweets and Spices 3126 Los Feliz Blvd., Los Angeles, CA 90039, 323-345-0360 *(WALK 26)*

Indochine Vien 3110 Glendale Blvd., Los Angeles, CA 90039, 323-667-9591 *(WALK 26)*

Intelligentsia Coffee and Tea 3922 W. Sunset Blvd., Los Angeles, CA 90026, 323-663-6173 *(WALK 27)*

J.J.'s Cafe 3599 Hayden Ave., Culver City, CA 90232, 310-837-3248 *(WALK 7)*

Joe's Restaurant 1023 Abbot Kinney Blvd., Venice, CA 90291, 310-399-5811 *(WALK 4)*

Kyoto Grand Hotel and Gardens 120 S. Los Angeles St., Los Angeles, CA 90012, 213-629-1200 *(WALK 32)*

La Ballona 3843 Main St., Culver City, CA 90232, 310-838-7409 *(WALK 8)*

LA Bread 3119 Los Feliz Blvd., Los Angeles, CA 90039, 323-662-8600 *(WALK 26)*

La Dijonaise 8703 Washington Blvd., Culver City, CA 90232, 310-287-2770 *(WALK 7)*

La Poubelle 5907 Franklin Ave., Los Angeles, CA 90028, 323-465-0807 *(WALK 18)*

Le Petit Greek 127 N. Larchmont Blvd., Los Angeles, CA 90004, 323-464-5160 *(WALK 21)*

Leimert Park Village Farmers Market Vision Theatre parking lot on the southeast corner of 43rd St. and Degnan Blvd., Los Angeles, CA 90008, Saturdays 10 A.M. to 3 P.M. *(WALK 9)*

Lilly's 1031 Abbot Kinney Blvd., Venice, CA 90291, 310-314-0004 *(WALK 4)*

Lucy Florence Coffee House and Le Florence Gallery 3351 W. 43rd St., Los Angeles, CA 90008, 323-293-1356 *(WALK 9)*

M&M Soul Food Restaurant 4317 Degnan Blvd., Los Angeles, CA 90008, 323-298-9898 *(WALK 9)*

Madame Matisse 3536 W. Sunset Blvd., Los Angeles, CA 90026, 323-662-4862 *(WALK 27)*

Mani's Bakery 519 S. Fairfax Ave., Los Angeles, CA 90036, 323-938-8800 *(WALK 14)*

McCormick & Schmick's 633 W. 5th St., Los Angeles, CA 90071, 213-629-1929 *(WALK 34)*

Mel's Drive-In 8585 W. Sunset Blvd., West Hollywood, CA 90069, 310-854-7200 *(WALK 12)*

Mexico City 2121 Hillhurst Ave., Los Angeles, CA 90027, 323-661-7227 *(WALK 23)*

Michelangelo Pizzeria Ristorante 1637 Silver Lake Blvd., Los Angeles, CA 90026, 323-660-4843 *(WALK 28)*

Mike & Anne's 1040 Mission St., South Pasadena, CA 91030, 626-799-7199 *(WALK 38)*

Millie's 3524 W. Sunset Blvd., Los Angeles, CA 90026, 323-664-0404 *(WALK 27)*

Mission Wines 1114 Mission St., South Pasadena, CA 91030, 626-403-9463 *(WALK 38)*

Miyagi's 8225 W. Sunset Blvd., West Hollywood, CA 90046, 323-650-3524 *(WALK 12)*

Mountain Bar 475 Gin Ling Way, Los Angeles, CA 90012, 213-625-7500 *(WALK 31)*

Musso & Frank Grill 6667 Hollywood Blvd., Los Angeles, CA 90028, 323-467-7788 *(WALK 17)*

Nicole's Gourmet Foods 921 Meridian Ave. Ste. B, South Pasadena, CA 91030, 626-403-5751 *(WALK 38)*

Novecento 3837 Main St., Culver City, CA 90232, 310-842-3838 *(WALK 8)*

Opus Bar & Grill 3760 Wilshire Blvd., Los Angeles, CA 90010, 213-738-1600 *(WALK 22)*

Palermo Italian Restaurant 1858 N. Vermont Ave., Los Angeles, CA 90027, 323-663-1178 *(WALK 23)*

Pazzo Gelato 3827 W. Sunset Blvd., Los Angeles, CA 90026, 323-662-1710 *(WALK 27)*

Philippe the Original 1001 N. Alameda St., Los Angeles, CA 90012, 213-628-3781 *(WALK 31)*

Phillip's BBQ 4307 Leimert Blvd., Los Angeles, CA 90008, 323-292-7613 *(WALK 9)*

Pig n' Whistle 6714 Hollywood Blvd., Los Angeles, CA 90028, 323-463-0000 *(WALK 17)*

Pinkberry 868 Huntley Dr., West Hollywood, CA 90069, 310-659-8285 *(WALK 13)*

Pit Fire Pizza Company 108 W. 2nd St., Los Angeles, CA 90012, 213-808-1200 *(WALK 33)*

Pit Fire Pizza Company 5108 Lankershim Blvd., North Hollywood, CA 91601, 818-980-2949 *(WALK 10)*

Poquito Mas 8555 W. Sunset Blvd., West Hollywood, CA 90069, 310-652-7008 *(WALK 12)*

Porch Restaurant 8430 W. Sunset Blvd., West Hollywood, CA 90069, 323-848-5100 *(WALK 12)*

Prado Restaurant 244 N. Larchmont Blvd., Los Angeles, CA 90004, 323-467-3871 *(WALK 21)*

Psychobabble 1866 N. Vermont Ave., Los Angeles, CA 90027, 323-664-7500 *(WALK 23)*

Real Raw Live 5913 Franklin Ave., Los Angeles, CA 90028, 323-461-4545 *(WALK 18)*

Roost 3100 Los Feliz Blvd., Los Angeles, CA 90039, 323-664-7272 *(WALK 26)*

Saddle Ranch Chop House 8371 W. Sunset Blvd., West Hollywood, CA 90069, 323-656-2007 *(WALK 12)*

Santa Maria Barbecue 9739 Culver Blvd., Culver City, CA 90232, 310-842-8169 *(WALK 8)*

Stroh's Gourmet 1239 Abbot Kinney Blvd., Venice, CA 90291, 310-450-5119 *(WALK 4)*

Sunny's Spot Coffee House 3349 W 43rd Pl., Los Angeles, CA 90008, 323-291-4075 *(WALK 9)*

Sweet Lady Jane 8360 Melrose Ave., West Hollywood, CA 90069, 323-653-7145 *(WALK 13)*

Tacos Villa Corona 3185 Glendale Blvd., Los Angeles, CA 90039, 323-661-3458 *(WALK 26)*

Taiyo Sushi 5917 Franklin Ave., Los Angeles, CA 90028, 323-468-2496 *(WALK 18)*

Tam O'Shanter 2980 Los Feliz Blvd., Los Angeles, CA 90039, 323-664-0228 *(WALK 26)*

Tangiers Lounge 2138 Hillhurst Ave., Los Angeles, CA 90027, 323-666-8666 *(WALK 23)*

Tender Greens 9523 Culver Blvd., Culver City, CA 90232, 310-842-8300 *(WALK 8)*

Tortilla Grill 1357 Abbot Kinney Blvd., Venice, CA 90291, 310-581-9953 *(WALK 4)*

Tokyo Delve's Sushi Bar 5239 Lankershim Blvd., North Hollywood, CA 91601, 818-766-3868 *(WALK 10)*

Traxx 800 N. Alameda St. (inside Union Station), Los Angeles, CA 90012, 213-625-1999 *(WALK 31)*

Urth Caffe 8565 Melrose Ave., West Hollywood, CA 90069, 310-659-0628 *(WALK 13)*

Utros Cafe Berth 73, San Pedro, CA 90731, 310-547-5022 *(WALK 36)*

Venice Farmers Market Corner of Dell Ave. and South Venice Blvd., Venice, CA 90291, Fridays 7 A.M. to 11 A.M. *(WALK 4)*

Vermont Restaurant and Bar 1714 N. Vermont Ave., Los Angeles, CA 90027, 323-661-6163 *(WALK 23)*

Village Coffee Shop 2695 N. Beachwood Dr., Los Angeles, CA 90068, 323-467-5398 *(WALK 19)*

Village French Bakery 1414 W. Kenneth Rd., Glendale, CA 91201, 818-241-2521 *(WALK 25)*

Village Pizzeria 131 N. Larchmont Blvd., Los Angeles, CA 90004, 323-465-5566 *(WALK 21)*

Vitello's Italian Restaurant 4349 Tujunga Ave., Studio City, CA 91604, 818-769-0905 *(WALK 11)*

Wahoo's Fish Taco 6258 Wilshire Blvd., Los Angeles, CA 90048, 323-933-2480 *(WALK 15)*

Wilshire Center Farmers Market Mariposa Ave. just north of Wilshire Blvd., Los Angeles, CA 90005, Fridays 11 A.M. to 3 P.M. *(WALK 22)*

Yamashiro 1999 N. Sycamore Ave., Los Angeles, CA 90068, 323-466-5125 *(WALK 17)*

HOTELS

Chateau Marmont 8221 W. Sunset Blvd., West Hollywood, CA 90046, 323-656-1010 *(WALK 12)*

Culver Hotel 9400 Culver Blvd., Culver City, CA 90232, 888-328-5837 *(WALK 8)*

Millennium Biltmore Hotel 506 S. Grand Ave., Los Angeles, CA 90071, 213-624-1011 *(WALK 34)*

Omni Hotel 251 S. Olive St., Los Angeles, CA 90012, 213-671-3300 *(WALK 33)*

Standard Hotel 8300 W. Sunset Blvd., West Hollywood, CA 90069, 323-650-9090 *(WALK 12)*

Sunset Tower Hotel 8358 W. Sunset Blvd., West Hollywood, CA 90069, 323-654-7100 *(WALK 12)*

Westin Bonaventure Hotel 404 S. Figueroa St., Los Angeles, CA 90071, 213-624-1000 *(WALK 34)*

ENTERTAINMENT AND NIGHTLIFE

Avery Schreiber Theatre 11050 Magnolia Blvd., North Hollywood, CA 91601, 818-761-0704 *(WALK 10)*

Babe's & Ricky's Inn 4339 Leimert Blvd., Los Angeles, CA 90008, 323-295-9112 *(WALK 9)*

Comedy Store 8433 W. Sunset Blvd., West Hollywood, CA 90069, 323-656-6225 *(WALK 12)*

Deaf West Theatre 5112 Lankershim Blvd., North Hollywood, CA 91601, 818-762-2998 *(WALK 10)*

Derby 4500 Los Feliz Blvd., Los Angeles, CA 90027, 323-663-8979 *(WALK 23)*

Egyptian Theatre 6712 Hollywood Blvd., Hollywood, CA 90028, 323-466-3456 *(WALK 17)*

El Capitan Theatre 6838 Hollywood Blvd., Los Angeles, CA 90068, 323-467-7674 *(WALK 17)*

El Portal Theatre 5269 Lankershim Blvd., North Hollywood, CA 91601, 213-480-3232 *(WALK 10)*

Grauman's Chinese Theatre 6925 Hollywood Blvd., Hollywood, CA 90028, 323-464-6266 *(WALK 17)*

House of Blues 8430 W. Sunset Blvd., West Hollywood, CA 90069, 323-848-5100 *(WALK 12)*

Jazz Bakery 3233 Helms Ave., Culver City, CA 90034, 310-271-9039 *(WALK 7)*

Kodak Theatre 6801 Hollywood Blvd., Los Angeles, CA 90028, 323-308-6300 *(WALK 17)*

Los Feliz 3 1822 N. Vermont Ave., Los Angeles, CA 90027, 323-664-2169 *(WALK 23)*

Magic Castle 7001 Franklin Ave., Los Angeles, CA 90068, 323-851-0800 *(WALK 17)*

Music Center (Dorothy Chandler Pavilion, Ahmanson Theatre, Mark Taper Forum) 135 N. Grand Ave., Los Angeles, CA 90012, 213-972-7211 *(WALK 33)*

NoHo Arts Center 11136 Magnolia Blvd., North Hollywood, CA 91601, 866-811-4111 *(WALK 10)*

Pantages Theatre 6233 Hollywood Blvd., Los Angeles, CA 90028, 323-468-1770 *(WALK 17)*
Regency West Theatre 3339 W. 43rd St., Los Angeles, CA 90008, 323-292-5143 *(WALK 9)*
Spaceland 1717 Silver Lake Blvd., Los Angeles, CA 90026, 213-833-2843 *(WALK 28)*
Two Roads Theatre 4348 Tujunga Ave., Studio City, CA 91604, 818-762-7488 *(WALK 10)*
Upright Citizens Brigade Theater 5919 Franklin Ave., Los Angeles, CA 90028, 323-908-8702 *(WALK 18)*
Walt Disney Concert Hall 111 S. Grand Ave., Los Angeles, CA 90012, 213-972-7211 *(WALK 33)*
Warner Grand Theatre 478 W. 6th St., San Pedro, CA 90731, 310-548-7672 *(WALK 10)*
Wiltern Theatre 3790 Wilshire Blvd., Los Angeles, CA 90010, 213-380-5005 *(WALK 22)*
World Stage Performance Gallery 4344 Degnan Blvd., Los Angeles, CA 90008, 323-293-2451 *(WALK 9)*

MUSEUMS aND GaLLeRies

American Heritage Masonic Museum 4357 Wilshire Blvd., Los Angeles, CA 90010, 323-930-9806
  (WALK 21)
Bergamot Station 2525 Michigan Ave., Santa Monica, CA 90404, 310-829-5854 *(WALK 3)*
California African American Museum 600 State Dr., Los Angeles, CA 90037, 213-744-7432 *(WALK 35)*
California Science Center 700 State Dr., Los Angeles, CA 90037, 323-724-3623
  or 213-744-7400 for IMAX Theater *(WALK 35)*
Erotic Museum 6741 Hollywood Blvd., Hollywood, CA 90028, 323-463-7684 *(WALK 17)*
Frederick's of Hollywood Lingerie Museum 6608 Hollywood Blvd., Hollywood, CA 90028, 323-466-8506
  (WALK 17)
Geffen Contemporary 152 N. Central Ave., Los Angeles, CA 90013, 213-621-2766 *(WALK 32)*
Hollywood Bowl Museum 2301 N. Highland Ave., Los Angeles CA 90068, 323-850-2058 *(WALK 16)*
Hollywood Heritage Museum 2100 N. Highland Ave., Los Angeles, CA 90068, 323-874-4005 *(WALK 16)*
Japanese American National Museum 369 E. 1st St., Los Angeles, CA 90012, 213-625-0414 *(WALK 32)*
Lankershim Arts Center 5108 Lankershim Blvd., North Hollywood, CA 91601, 818-760-1278 *(WALK 10)*
Los Angeles County Museum of Art 5905 Wilshire Blvd., Los Angeles, CA 90036, 323-857-6000
  (WALK 14)
Los Angeles Maritime Museum Berth 84 (foot of 6th St.), San Pedro, CA 90731, 310-548-7618 *(WALK 36)*
Lowe Gallery 2034 Broadway Blvd., Santa Monica, CA 90404, 310-449-0184 *(WALK 3)*
Museum of Contemporary Art 250 S. Grand Ave., Los Angeles, CA 90012, 213-626-6222 *(WALK 33)*
Natural History Museum 900 Exposition Blvd., Los Angeles, CA 90007, 213-763-3466 *(WALK 35)*
Pacific Design Center 8687 Melrose Ave., West Hollywood, CA 90068, 310-657-0800 *(WALK 13)*
Page Museum 5801 Wilshire Blvd., Los Angeles, CA 90036, 323-934-7243 *(WALK 14)*

Schindler House and MAK Center for Design 835 N. Kings Rd., West Hollywood, CA 90068, 323-651-1510 *(WALK 13)*

South Pasadena Historical Museum 913 Meridian St., South Pasadena, CA 91030, 626-799-9089 *(WALK 38)*

educational and cultural centers

Brand Library & Art Center 1601 W. Mountain St., Glendale, CA 91201, 818-548-2051 *(WALK 25)*

Central Library 630 W. 5th St., Los Angeles, CA 90071, 213-228-7000 *(WALK 34)*

Japanese American Cultural and Community Center 244 S. San Pedro St. Ste. 505, Los Angeles, CA 90012, 213-628-2725 *(WALK 32)*

Historical landmarks and monuments

Avila Adobe 10 Olvera St., Los Angeles, CA 90012, 213-628-1274 *(WALK 31)*

Barnsdall Art Park/Hollyhock House 4800 Hollywood Blvd., Los Angeles, CA 90027, 323-644-6269 *(WALK 23)*

City Hall 200 N. Spring St., Los Angeles, CA 90012, 213-473-7001 *(WALK 33)*

Ebell Club of Los Angeles 743 S. Lucerne Blvd., Los Angeles, CA 90005, 323-931-1277 *(WALK 21)*

Ennis-Brown House 2607 Glendower Ave., Los Angeles, CA 90027, 323-668-0234 *(WALK 23)*

Firehouse No. 1 134 Paseo de la Plaza, Los Angeles, CA 90012, 213-628-1274 *(WALK 31)*

Los Angeles Theatre 615 S. Broadway, Los Angeles CA 90014, 213-629-2939 *(WALK 34)*

spiritual institutions

Cathedral of Our Lady of Angels 555 W. Temple St., Los Angeles, CA 90012, 213-680-5200 *(WALK 33)*

Lake Shrine Temple 17190 Sunset Blvd., Pacific Palisades, CA 90272, 310-454-4114 *(WALK 1)*

Self-Realization Fellowship 3880 San Rafael Dr., Los Angeles, CA 90065, 323-225-2471 *(WALK 37)*

St. Basil's Catholic Church 3611 Wilshire Blvd., Los Angeles, CA 90010, 213-382-6337 *(WALK 22)*

Vedanta Society of Southern California 1946 Vedanta Pl., Hollywood, CA 90068, 323-465-7114 *(WALK 18)*

Wilshire Boulevard Temple 3663 Wilshire Blvd., Los Angeles, CA 90010, 213-388-2401 *(WALK 22)*

Wilshire Christian Church 634 S. Normandie Ave., Los Angeles, CA 90005, 213-382-6337 *(WALK 22)*

SHOPPING

Abuelita's 1012 Mission St., South Pasadena, CA 91030, 626-799-0355 *(WALK 38)*

Audrey K. 1411½ W. Kenneth Rd., Glendale, CA 91201, 818-242-5758 *(WALK 25)*

Bodhi Tree Bookstore 8585 Melrose Ave., West Hollywood, CA 90069, 310-659-1733 *(WALK 13)*

Book 'Em Mysteries 1118 Mission St., South Pasadena, CA 91030, 626-799-9600 *(WALK 38)*

Book Soup 8818 W. Sunset Blvd., West Hollywood, CA 90069, 310-659-3110 *(WALK 12)*

Counterpoint Records & Books 5911 Franklin Ave., Los Angeles, CA 90028, 323-957-7965 *(WALK 18)*

Den of Antiquity 3902 W. Sunset Blvd., Los Angeles, CA 90027, 323-666-3881 *(WALK 27)*

Dinosaur Farm 1510 Mission St., South Pasadena, CA 91030, 626-441-2767 *(WALK 38)*

Eso Won Books 4331 Degnan Blvd., Los Angeles, CA 90008, 323-290-1048 *(WALK 9)*

The Grove 189 The Grove Dr., Los Angeles, CA 90036, 888-315-8883 *(WALK 14)*

H.D. Buttercup 3225 Helms Ave., Culver City, CA 90034, 310-558-8900 *(WALK 7)*

Heritage Bookshop 8540 Melrose Ave., West Hollywood, CA 90069, 310-659-3674 *(WALK 13)*

Hollywood & Highland 6801 Hollywood Blvd., Los Angeles, 90028, 323-960-2331 *(WALK 17)*

Hollywood Toys & Costumes 6600 Hollywood Blvd., Hollywood, CA 90028, 323-464-4444 *(WALK 17)*

Ivy's Flower Station 1435 W. Kenneth Rd., Glendale, CA 91201, 818-500-7599 *(WALK 25)*

Livin' Art 1130 Mission St., South Pasadena, CA 91030, 626-799-8278 *(WALK 38)*

Organic Rush 960 Mission St., South Pasadena, CA 91030, 626-799-8099 *(WALK 38)*

Pet Rush 1420 W. Kenneth Rd. Glendale, CA 91201, 818-956-0029 *(WALK 25)*

Potted 3158 Los Feliz Blvd., Los Angeles, CA 90039, 323-665-3801 *(WALK 26)*

Pull My Daisy 3908 W. Sunset Blvd., Los Angeles, CA 90029, 323-663-0608 *(WALK 27)*

Retro Parc 1405 W. Kenneth Rd., Glendale, CA 91201, 818-242-3104 *(WALK 25)*

Rubbish 1627 Silver Lake Blvd., Los Angeles, CA 90026, 323-661-5575 *(WALK 28)*

Skylight Books 1818 N. Vermont Ave., Los Angeles, CA 90027, 323-660-1175 *(WALK 23)*

Squaresville 1800 N. Vermont Ave., Los Angeles, CA 90027, 323-669-8464 *(WALK 23)*

Surplus Value Center 3828 W. Sunset Blvd., Los Angeles, CA 90026, 323-662-8132 *(WALK 27)*

Williams Bookstore 443 W. 6th St., San Pedro, CA 90731, 310-832-3631 *(WALK 36)*

Wing Hop Fung Ginseng and China Products Center 727 N. Broadway, Los Angeles, CA 90012, 213-626-7200 *(WALK 31)*

Yolk 1626 Silver Lake Blvd., Los Angeles, CA 90026, 323-660-4315 *(WALK 28)*

Zambezi Bazaar 4334 Degnan Blvd., Los Angeles, CA 90008, 323-299-6383 *(WALK 9)*

Beauty and Health

Aroma Spa and Sports 3680 Wilshire Blvd., Los Angeles, CA 90010, 213-387-0212 *(WALK 22)*

Being in LA 2016 Hillhurst Ave., Los Angeles, CA 90027, 323-665-9355 *(WALK 23)*

Brooks Massage Therapy 7619-21 Beverly Blvd., Los Angeles, CA 90036, 323-937-8781 *(WALK 14)*

Dr. Tea's Tea Garden & Herbal Emporium 8612 Melrose Ave., West Hollywood, CA 90069, 310-657-9300 *(WALK 13)*

dtox Day Spa 3206 Los Feliz Blvd., Los Angeles, CA 90039, 323-665-3869 *(WALK 26)*

Karuna Yoga 1939½ Hillhurst Ave., Los Angeles, CA 90027, 323-665-6242 *(WALK 23)*

Larchmont Beauty Center 208 N. Larchmont Blvd., Los Angeles, CA 90004, 323-461-0162 *(WALK 21)*

Massage Garage 3812 Main St., Culver City, CA 90232, 310-202-0082 *(WALK 8)*

Massage Place and Petit Spa 625 Montana Ave., Santa Monica, CA 90403, 310-393-7007 *(WALK 2)*

Mission Street Yoga 1017 Mission St., South Pasadena, CA 91030, 626-441-1144 *(WALK 38)*

Puff 1005 Mission St., South Pasadena, CA 91030, 626-799-2864 *(WALK 38)*

Spoiled: A Day Spa 4338 Tujunga Ave., Studio City, CA 91604, 818-508-9772 *(WALK 11)*

Parks and Gardens

Exposition Park Rose Garden 701 State Dr., Los Angeles, CA 90037, 213-763-0114 *(WALK 35)*

La Cienega Park Community Center 8400 Gregory Way, Beverly Hills, CA 90211, 310-550-4625 *(WALK 15)*

Mildred E. Mathias Botanical Garden University of California, Los Angeles, Los Angeles, CA 90095, 310-825-1260 *(WALK 6)*

Pan Pacific Regional Park 7600 Beverly Blvd., Los Angeles, CA 90036, 323-939-8874 *(WALK 14)*

Silver Lake Recreation Center 1850 Silver Lake Blvd., Los Angeles, CA 90026, 323-644-3946 *(WALK 28)*

Westminster Off-Leash Dog Park 1234 Pacific Ave., Venice, CA 90291, 310-301-1550 *(WALK 4)*

William S. Hart Park 8341 De Longpre Ave., West Hollywood, CA 90069, 323-848-6308 *(WALK 12)*

miscellaneous

Academy of Television Arts and Sciences 5220 Lankershim Blvd., North Hollywood, CA 91601,
   818-754-2800 *(WALK 10)*

Los Angeles Memorial Coliseum 3911 S. Figueroa St., Los Angeles, CA 90037, 213-747-7111 *(WALK 35)*

Los Feliz Municipal Golf Course 3207 Los Feliz Blvd., Los Angeles, CA 90039, 323-663-7758 *(WALK 26)*

Lovecraft Biofuels 4000 W. Sunset Blvd., Los Angeles, CA 90029, 323-644-9072 *(WALK 27)*

Sony Pictures Studios 10202 West Washington Blvd., Culver City, CA 90232, 323-520-TOUR *(WALK 8)*

APPENDIX 3: Calories Burned Per Walk

Calorie estimates are based on the duration of the walk and the approximate rate at which individuals of given weights burn calories at each speed.

Walk		CALORIES BURNED AT 2.5 MPH				
		110–130 lbs	130–150 lbs	150–170 lbs	170–200 lbs	200–230 lbs
1.	Castellammare	75–88	88–102	102–116	116–136	136–156
2.	Northwest Santa Monica	120–142	142–163	163–185	185–218	218–250
3.	Southeast Santa Monica	60–71	71–82	82–93	93–109	109–125
4.	Venice Beach	120–142	142–163	163–185	185–218	218–250
5.	Mar Vista	45–53	53–61	61–69	69–82	82–94
6.	UCLA Campus	105–124	124–143	143–162	162–191	191–219
7.	North Culver City	90–106	106–122	122–139	139–163	163–188
8.	Downtown Culver City	210–248	248–286	286–324	324–381	381–438
9.	Leimert Park Village	27–32	32–37	37–42	42–49	49–56
10.	NoHo Arts District	45–53	53–61	61–69	69–82	82–94
11.	Studio City's Woodbridge Park	90–106	106–122	122–139	139–163	163–188
12.	Sunset Strip	150–177	177–204	204–231	213–272	272–313
13.	West Hollywood	120–142	142–163	163–185	185–218	218–250
14.	Miracle Mile	150–177	177–204	204–231	231–272	272–313
15.	Carthay Circle & South Carthay	120–142	142–163	163–185	185–218	218–250
16.	High Tower & the Hollywood Bowl	60–71	71–82	82–93	93–109	109–125
17.	Whitley Heights & Hollywood Blvd.	120–142	142–163	163–185	185–218	218–250
18.	Lower Beachwood Canyon	120–142	142–163	163–185	185–218	218–250
19.	Upper Beachwood Canyon	120–142	142–163	163–185	185–218	218–250
20.	Melrose Hill	30–35	35–41	41–46	46–54	54–63

CALORIES BURNED AT 3.5 MPH

110–130 lbs	130–150 lbs	150–170 lbs	170–200 lbs	200–230 lbs
68–80	80–92	92–105	105–123	123–142
108–128	128–148	148–167	167–197	197–227
54–64	64–74	74–84	84–98	98–113
108–128	128–148	148–167	167–197	197–227
41–48	48–55	55–63	63–74	74–85
95–112	112–129	129–147	147–172	172–198
81–96	96–111	111–126	126–148	148–170
190–224	224–259	259–293	293–345	345–396
24–29	29–33	33–38	38–44	44–51
41–48	48–55	55–63	63–74	74–85
81–96	96–111	111–126	126–148	148–170
135–160	160–185	185–209	209–246	246–283
108–128	128–148	148–167	167–197	197–227
135–160	160–185	185–209	209–246	246–283
108–128	128–148	148–167	167–197	197–227
54–64	64–74	74–84	84–98	98–113
108–128	128–148	148–167	167–197	197–227
108–128	128–148	148–167	167–197	197–227
108–128	128–148	148–167	167–197	197–227
27–32	32–37	37–42	42–49	49–57

CALORIES BURNED AT 2.5 MPH

Walk	110–130 lbs	130–150 lbs	150–170 lbs	170–200 lbs	200–230 lbs
21. Larchmont Village & Windsor Square	120–142	142–163	163–185	185–218	218–250
22. Koreatown/Wilshire Center	90–106	106–122	122–139	139–163	163–188
23. Los Feliz	90–106	106–122	122–139	139–163	163–188
Los Feliz with Addendum	210–248	248–286	286–324	324–381	381–438
24. Franklin Hills	30–35	35–41	41–46	46–54	54–63
25. Brand Park & Kenneth Village	90–106	106–122	122–139	139–163	162–188
26. Atwater Village	120–142	142–163	163–185	185–218	218–250
27. West Silver Lake	105–124	124–143	143–162	162–191	191–219
28. East Silver Lake	120–142	142–163	163–185	185–218	218–250
29. Echo Park & Angelino Heights	120–142	142–163	163–185	185–218	218–250
30. Elysian Heights	45–53	53–61	61–69	69–82	82–94
31. El Pueblo de Los Angeles & Chinatown	120–142	142–163	163–185	185–218	218–250
32. Little Tokyo	45–53	53–61	61–69	69–82	82–94
33. Downtown Civic Center	120–142	142–163	163–185	185–218	218–250
34. Downtown Financial & Jewelry Districts	90–106	106–122	122–139	139–163	163–188
35. USC & Exposition Park	90–106	106–122	122–139	139–163	163–188
36. San Pedro	120–142	142–163	163–185	185–218	218–250
37. Mt. Washington	15–18	18–20	20–23	23–27	27–31
Mt. Washington with Addendum	90–106	106–122	122–139	139–163	163–188
38. South Pasadena	61–71	71–82	82–93	93–109	109–125

CALORIES BURNED AT 3.5 MPH

110–130 lbs	130–150 lbs	150–170 lbs	170–200 lbs	200–230 lbs
108–128	128–148	148–167	167–197	197–227
81–96	96–111	111–126	126–148	148–170
81–96	96–111	111–126	126–148	148–170
190–224	224–259	259–293	293–345	345–396
27–32	32–37	37–42	42–49	49–57
81–91	96–111	111–126	126–148	148–170
108–128	128–148	148–167	167–197	197–227
95–112	112–129	129–147	147–172	172–198
108–128	128–148	148–167	167–197	197–227
108–128	128–148	148–167	167–197	197–227
41–48	48–55	55–63	63–74	74–85
108–128	128–148	148–167	167–197	197–227
41–48	48–55	55–63	63–74	74–85
108–128	128–148	148–167	167–197	197–227
81–96	96–111	111–126	126–148	148–170
81–96	96–111	111–126	126–148	148–170
108–128	128–148	148–167	167–197	197–227
14–16	16–18	18–21	21–25	25–28
81–96	96–111	111–126	126–148	148–170
54–64	64–74	74–84	84–98	98–113

INDEX

(*Italicized* page numbers indicate photos.)

about the author

Southern California native Erin Mahoney Harris loves to walk, yet she's lived most of her life in areas that wouldn't typically be considered pedestrian-friendly. Undaunted, she makes it a point to hoof it whenever possible. She finds walking to be meditative, invigorating, and almost always rewarding, as there are so many fascinating features and landmarks in Los Angeles that are easy to miss when whizzing by in a car.

Erin is the founder and editor of ChillOutLA.com, a guide to health, beauty, and relaxation deals in Los Angeles. She currently lives in the Hollywood Hills with her husband, Tony, her son, West, and her Golden Retriever/Chow mix, Tuffy.

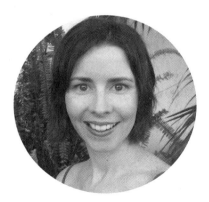

TaKe an urBan TreK
WITH a BOOK From THe
award-WINNING WaLKING series!

The WaLKING books are a must for the inquisitive urban adventurer, whether you're a local discovering your city with fresh eyes, or a visitor seeking a more authentic travel experience. Each tour in this stylish series features history, culture, and local architecture, plus recommendations on eateries, galleries, and nightlife. With detailed maps, parking and public transit information, at-a-glance walk highlights, and contact information for hundreds of points of interest, there's no better way to discover a city than on foot with a WaLKING guide.

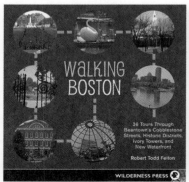

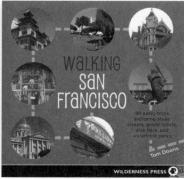

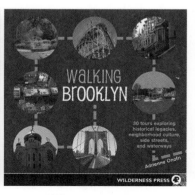

ISBN 978-0-89997-448-4

ISBN 978-0-89997-419-4

ISBN 978-0-89997-430-9